NEW DIRECTIONS FOR MENTAL HEALTH SERVICES

H. Richard Lamb, *University of Southern California*
EDITOR-IN-CHIEF

Deinstitutionalization: Promise and Problems

H. Richard Lamb
University of Southern California

Linda E. Weinberger
University of Southern California

EDITORS

Number 90, Summer 2001

JOSSEY-BASS
San Francisco

DEINSTITUTIONALIZATION: PROMISE AND PROBLEMS
H. Richard Lamb, Linda E. Weinberger (eds.)
New Directions for Mental Health Services, no. 90
H. Richard Lamb, Editor-in-Chief

Microfilm copies of issues and articles are available in 16mm and 35mm, as well as microfiche in 105mm, through University Microfilms Inc., 300 North Zeeb Road, Ann Arbor, Michigan 48106–1346.

ISSN 0193–9416   ISBN 0–7879–1439–8

NEW DIRECTIONS FOR MENTAL HEALTH SERVICES is part of The Jossey-Bass Psychology Series and is published quarterly by Jossey-Bass Inc., Publishers, 350 Sansome Street, San Francisco, California 94104-1342.

SUBSCRIPTIONS cost $66.00 for individuals and $121.00 for institutions, agencies, and libraries.

EDITORIAL CORRESPONDENCE should be sent to the Editor-in-Chief, H. Richard Lamb, University of Southern California, Department of Psychiatry, Graduate Hall, 1937 Hospital Place, Los Angeles, California 90033–1071.

Cover photograph by Wernher Krutein/PHOTOVAULT ©1990.

Jossey-Bass Web address: www.josseybass.com

Printed in the United States of America on acid-free recycled paper containing 100 percent recovered waste paper, of which at least 20 percent is postconsumer waste.

Contents

EDITORS' NOTES

Both the scope and effects of deinstitutionalization have been dramatic. For many years, we have combined our perspectives and expertise in public psychiatry and clinical forensic psychology to study and write about various aspects of deinstitutionalization. This volume examines both positive and negative effects of this mass movement of persons with severe mental illness out of the state hospitals and into the community. Although deinstitutionalization for most of this population can result in a much richer life experience in the community, much more needs to be done to make that occur.

The volume begins with an overview of the successes and disappointments of deinstitutionalization. Next, Chapter Two contains a study of the problems that result when the use of community alternatives to state hospitalization, often driven by lower costs and an ideology that highly structured care is seldom needed, is not adequate to meet the needs of these persons.

The next four chapters address one of the greatest problems of deinstitutionalization: the very large number of persons with severe mental illness who have found their way into the criminal justice system. Mental health professionals, families, the media, and society generally have become increasingly concerned about the number of persons with severe mental illness in jails and prisons. Why this has happened and what to do about it are the subjects of Chapter Three.

Chapter Four reviews community treatment of severely mentally ill offenders under the jurisdiction of the criminal justice system. In traditional treatment of persons with severe mental illness, the primary focus is usually on an alleviation of symptoms. However, treatment of members of this population who have committed crimes and must now comply with legal restrictions on their behavior must first address risk of harm to the community. In this effort, it is critical to identify a treatment philosophy that strikes a balance between individual rights and public safety and includes clear treatment goals, which the authors of this chapter describe in some detail.

Chapter Five reports on a study of a program that attempts to prevent inappropriate entry of mentally ill persons into the criminal justice system using outreach emergency teams comprising police officers and mental health professionals. These teams assess and make appropriate dispositions in the field of persons who have acute and severe mental illness, a high potential for violence, a high incidence of substance abuse, and long histories with both the criminal justice and mental health systems. Such teams are shown to be able to avoid criminalization of the mentally ill.

Another way to avoid criminalization is to provide mental health consultation to a municipal court and recommend court-mandated interventions

1

for mentally ill persons who have committed minor crimes. This is the subject of Chapter Six, which also demonstrates that when the judge both mandates and monitors mental health treatment, a significantly better outcome results.

Chapter Seven, on the therapeutic use of conservatorship with persons who have severe mental illness, describes how mental health conservatorship in California plays an important role in clinical management and treatment of mentally ill persons. The civil conservatorship process is a mechanism that allows for imposing sufficient structure on individuals who are not under the jurisdiction of the criminal justice system so they can live successfully in the community.

The final chapter turns to the subject of psychiatric rehabilitation. It outlines the broad historical developments and prominent current modalities and models of psychiatric rehabilitation: the introduction of family care, the day hospital, social skills training, psychoeducation, and the Fountain House model. The conceptual underpinnings of the field are discussed, including the need to work with the healthy part of the client's ego. The chapter concludes with an examination of some current issues in rehabilitation.

H. Richard Lamb
Linda E. Weinberger
Editors

H. RICHARD LAMB is professor of psychiatry and the behavioral sciences at Keck School of Medicine, University of Southern California, in Los Angeles.

LINDA E. WEINBERGER is professor of clinical psychiatry and chief psychologist at the Institute of Psychiatry, Law, and Behavioral Sciences at Keck School of Medicine, University of Southern California, in Los Angeles.

1 *This overview of deinstitutionalization explores its accomplishments and disappointments.*

Deinstitutionalization at the Beginning of the New Millennium

H. Richard Lamb

Among the milestones in the care and treatment of chronically and severely mentally ill persons in the second half of the twentieth century, deinstitutionalization (the mass exodus of mentally ill persons from living in hospitals to living in the community), the discovery of chlorpromazine and other modern antipsychotic medications, and the development of community psychosocial treatment and rehabilitation stand out. As British social psychiatrist John Wing (1990) has pointed out, deinstitutionalization and the use of psychosocial treatment were made possible on such a massive scale by the dramatic effects of these new medications on behavior and symptoms.

What has been learned from the successes and failures of deinstitutionalization? Over the past four decades, many things have been done well, and many mistakes have been made. This review examines both the positive and the negative aspects of this revolution in mental health care.

The dimensions of deinstitutionalization in the United States are impressive. In 1955, when numbers of patients in state hospitals reached their highest point, 559,000 persons were institutionalized in state mental hospitals out of a total national population of 165 million; in 1998 there were 57,151 for a population of more than 275 million (Survey and Analysis Branch, Center for Mental Health Services, 2000). Thus, in about forty years, the United States reduced its number of occupied state hospital beds from 339 per 100,000 population to twenty-one per 100,000 on any given day. Some states have gone even further. In California, for example, there are now only four state hospital beds, not including those set aside for forensic patients, per 100,000 population

Source: Lamb, H.R. "Deinstitutionalization at the Beginning of the New Millennium." *Harvard Review of Psychiatry*, 1998, 6, 1–9. Reprinted by permission.

(John Rodriguez, California State Department of Mental Health, personal communication, 1997).

A Primary Problem of Deinstitutionalization

Much of the concern about deinstitutionalization has focused on the fate of patients discharged into the community after many years of hospitalization. However, the problem that has proved most vexing—the treatment of the new generation that has grown up since deinstitutionalization—was almost totally unforeseen by the advocates of deinstitutionalization. Today's homeless mentally ill are primarily from this new generation (Hopper, Baxter, and Cox, 1982). The large homeless population with major mental illness (schizophrenia, schizoaffective disorder, bipolar illness, or major depression with psychotic features) has tended to be young.

How did this come to be? The majority of the current long-stay hospitalized patients who are most inappropriate for discharge, because of a propensity to physical violence, very poor coping skills, or a marked degree of manifest pathology, will not be discharged, or if they are discharged and fail, they will not be sent out again.

Persons who have been hospitalized for long periods have been institutionalized to passivity (Lamb, 1993). For the most part, they have come to do what they are told. When those for whom discharge from the hospital is feasible and appropriate are placed in a community living situation with sufficient support and structure, most (although by no means all) tend to stay where they are placed and to accept treatment.

This sequence has not been true for the new generation of severely mentally ill persons. They have not been institutionalized to passivity. Not only have they not spent long years in hospitals, but they have probably had difficulty just getting admitted to an acute hospital (whether they wanted to be or not) and even greater difficulty staying there for more than a short period on any one admission.

Taking an Existential Perspective

To understand the plight of this new generation of the chronically and severely mentally ill, we should consider their problems from an existential point of view. There is evidence that chronically and severely mentally ill persons have fewer goals to make changes in their lives as they move into their thirties. For instance, a study of severely disabled psychiatric patients in a board-and-care home (Lamb, 1979) showed that compared to patients under age thirty, significantly fewer patients age thirty and older had goals to change anything in their lives. How can we understand this finding? Perhaps as these persons have become older, they have had more time to experience repeated failures in dealing with life's demands and achieving their earlier goals. They have had more time to lower or set aside their goals and to accept a life with a level of functioning that does not exceed their limited capabilities. In the same study, a strong relationship was found between age and history of hospitalization: 74 percent of patients under age thirty had been hospitalized during the preceding year as compared to only 21 percent of those age thirty and older.

When one is still young and has just begun to deal with life's demands and is trying to make one's way in the world, one struggles to achieve some measure of independence, to choose and succeed at a vocation, to establish satisfying interpersonal relationships and attain some degree of intimacy, and to acquire a sense of identity. Absent the abilities to withstand stress and to form meaningful interpersonal relationships, the mentally ill person's efforts often lead to failure. The result may be a yet-more-determined—often frantic—effort with a greatly increased level of anxiety, even desperation. Ultimately, this may lead to another failure, accompanied by feelings of despair. For a person predisposed to decompensate under stress, the course is predictably stormy, with acute psychotic breaks and repeated hospitalizations, often related to these desperate attempts to achieve (Lamb, 1982a). The situation becomes even worse when such individuals are in an environment where unrealistic expectations emanate not just from within themselves, but also from families and mental health professionals.

Before deinstitutionalization these "new" chronic patients would have been institutionalized for lengthy periods, often starting from the time of their first break in adolescence or early childhood. Sometimes such patients recompensated in the hospital and were discharged, but at the point of their next decompensation they were rehospitalized, often never to return to the community. Thus, following their initial failures in trying to cope with the vicissitudes of life and living in the community, these persons were no longer exposed to such stresses; they were given permanent asylum from the demands of the world. Unfortunately, the ways in which state hospitals achieved this structure and asylum led to everyday abuses that left scars on the mental health professions, as well as on the patients. Today, however, hospital stays tend to be brief.

In this sense, the majority of "new" long-term patients are the products of deinstitutionalization. This is not to suggest that we should turn the clock back and return to a system of total institutionalization for all chronically mentally ill patients. In the community, most of these patients can have something very precious—their liberty, to the extent that they can handle it. Furthermore, if we provide the resources, they can realize their potential to attain some of life's milestones. Nevertheless, the plight of this new generation of chronically and severely mentally ill persons has occasioned many of the concerns about deinstitutionalization. Such persons have posed the most difficult clinical problems in treatment and have swollen the ranks of the homeless mentally ill and the mentally ill in jail. This has created serious social problems for society (Pepper, Kirshner, and Ryglewicz, 1981; Lamb, 1984; Lamb and Weinberger, 1998).

Problems in Treatment of the "New" Long-Term Patients

Less than half a century ago, there were no antipsychotic medications to bring chronically and severely mentally ill persons out of their world of delusional thoughts and help them return to the community. Even today, many patients fail to take psychotropic medications because of disturbing side effects, fear of tardive dyskinesia, or denial of illness. Van Putten, Crumpton, and Yale (1976) speculated that in some cases, patients do not take their medications in order to avoid the dysphoric feelings of depression and anxiety that result when they see their reality too clearly; grandiosity and a blurring of reality may make their lives more bearable than a relative, drug-induced normality.

The "new" chronic patients often deny a need for mental health treatment and eschew the identity of chronic mental patient (Minkoff, 1987). Admitting mental illness appears tantamount to conceding failure. Becoming part of the mental health system seems to many of these persons like joining an army of misfits (Lamb, 1982a). Significant numbers of these individuals also have primary substance abuse disorders or medicate themselves with street drugs, or both (Minkoff and Drake, 1991). Another factor contributing to refusal of treatment is the natural rebelliousness of youth.

Institutionalism

In the 1960s, social psychiatrist John Wing and sociologist George Brown (1970) observed that persons who spent long periods in mental hospitals developed what has come to be known as *institutionalism*, a syndrome characterized by lack of initiative, apathy, withdrawal, submissiveness to authority, and excessive dependence on the institution. Sociologists such as Erving Goffman (1961) argued that in what he called "total institutions" (for example, state mental hospitals), impersonal treatment can strip away a patient's dignity and individuality and foster regression; the "deviant" person is thus locked into a degraded, stigmatized, deviant role. Goffman and others believed that the social environment in institutions could strongly influence the emergence of psychotic symptoms and behavior. Other investigators (Johnstone and others, 1981), however, observed that institutionalism is probably not entirely the outcome of living in dehumanizing institutions; such characteristics may be linked to the schizophrenic process itself.

With deinstitutionalization, these latter researchers observed that many chronically and severely mentally ill persons who were vulnerable to institutionalism seemed to develop dependence on any way of life in the community that provided minimal social stimulation and allowed them to be socially inactive. They gravitated toward a lifestyle that permitted them to remain free from symptoms and painful and depressive feelings. In addition, the negative symptoms of schizophrenia may well have been playing a role here (Andreasen, 1982; Mueser, Douglas, Bellack, and Morrison, 1991).

Is this dependent, inactive lifestyle bad? For many deinstitutionalized persons, it may lead to unnecessary regression and impede social and vocational functioning. Such a lifestyle should thus be discouraged for these individuals so that they may realize their potential for higher community functioning. On the other hand, a restricted lifestyle may meet the needs of many deinstitutionalized severely mentally ill persons and help them to stay in the community. Mental health professionals and society at large are coming to recognize the crippling limitations of mental illness that in some cases do not yield to current treatment methods, including the latest generation of antipsychotic medications. It is important to provide adequate care for this vulnerable group so that the end result is not like the fate of the mentally ill in the back wards of state hospitals. For the patient who can be restored only to a degree, many mental health professionals advocate realistic expectations, responsibilities consistent with the person's potential, and providing reasonable comfort and, when indicated, an undemanding life with dignity (Dincin, 1995).

Some Basic Needs of Chronically and Severely Mentally Ill Persons in the Community

The experience with deinstitutionalization has made clear that a comprehensive and integrated system of care for the chronically and severely mentally ill, with designated responsibility, accountability, and adequate fiscal resources, needs to be established in the community (Talbott and Lamb, 1984). With such a system in place, patients' level of functioning and quality of life can be greatly enhanced. The following are the components of such a system.

Adequate, comprehensive, and accessible psychiatric and rehabilitative services need to be available and, when necessary, provided through outreach programs. Direct psychiatric services should provide outreach contact with the mentally ill in the community, psychiatric assessment and evaluation, crisis intervention (including hospitalization), individualized treatment plans, psychotropic medication and other somatic therapies, and psychosocial treatment. Rehabilitative services should include socialization experiences, training in the skills of everyday living, and social and vocational rehabilitation. Both treatment and rehabilitative services must be provided assertively (Stein, 1992)—for instance, by going out to patients' living settings if they do not or cannot come to a centralized program location.

Assertive community treatment has been shown to be effective in accomplishing many of these goals (Burns and Santos, 1995). In such programs multidisciplinary teams provide services directly to patients in the community. Staff work together closely in small teams, thus supplying single-point accountability for the care of individual patients and improving coordination and continuity of care. The teams respond to crises around the clock if need be, thus reducing the use of hospitalization. On a regular basis, they go to the patients wherever they are in the community and assist them in making adjustments to vocational, living, social, and recreational situations. Medication monitoring is another important function.

Crisis services need to be available and accessible. Too often, chronically and severely mentally ill persons who are in crisis situations are put into inpatient hospital units when rapid specific interventions, such as medication or emergency housing, would be more effective and less costly. This can cause others in need of acute hospitalization to be denied it because of shortages of hospital beds.

An adequate number and ample range of graded, stepwise, supervised community housing settings need to be established. Some chronically and severely mentally ill persons can graduate to fully independent living. For many, however, mainstream low-cost housing is not appropriate; housing settings that require people to manage entirely by themselves are beyond their capabilities (Talbott and Lamb, 1984). Instead, settings offering different levels of supervision, both more and less intensive, need to be available: halfway houses, board-and-care homes, supervised satellite apartment programs, foster or family care, and crisis or temporary hostels.

A system of responsibility for the chronically and severely mentally ill living in the community needs to be established, with the goal of ensuring that each patient has a therapeutic relationship with one mental health professional or paraprofessional (a case manager) who is ultimately responsible for his or her care. In such a system, each patient's case manager would ensure that the appropriate psychiatric and medical assessments were carried out; would formulate, together with the patient, an individualized treatment and rehabilitation plan, including the proper pharmacotherapy; would monitor the patient; and would assist the patient in receiving services.

Clearly, the shift of psychiatric care from institutional to community settings does not eliminate the necessity to continue the provision of comprehensive services to mentally ill persons. Consequently, society needs to declare a public policy of responsibility for the mentally ill who are unable to meet their own needs; governments need to designate and fund programs in each region or locale as core entities responsible and accountable for the care of the chronically and severely mentally ill living there; and the staff of these agencies need to be assigned individual patients for whom they are responsible.

For the chronically and severely mentally ill persons who live at home (currently more than 50 percent) or have positive ongoing relationships with their families, programs and respite care need to be provided to enhance the family's ability to provide a support system (Hatfield, 1994). Here the use of family systems is not feasible, and the mentally ill person needs to be linked with a formal community support system. In any case, the entire burden of deinstitutionalization should not be allowed to fall on families.

Basic changes need to be effected in legal and administrative procedures to ensure continuing community care for the chronically and severely mentally ill. In the 1960s and 1970s, a combination of laws that made commitment harder to obtain and patients' rights advocacy remedied some very serious abuses in public hospital care. At the same time, it became more difficult for many persons who need involuntary treatment to receive it (Lamb and Mills, 1986).

Involuntary commitment laws need to be made more humane to permit prompt return to active inpatient treatment for mentally ill persons when acute exacerbations of their illnesses make life in the community chaotic and unbearable. Treatment laws should allow (and facilitate, when necessary) the option of outpatient civil commitment, whereby the court mandates treatment at a mental health outpatient facility rather than ordering commitment to a hospital (Jemelka, Trupin, and Chiles, 1989; Hoffman, 1990; Swanson and others, 1997). In states that already have provisions for such treatment, the mechanism should be more widely used. Finally, advocacy efforts should be focused on the availability of effective care in the community rather than simply on "liberty" for mentally ill persons at any cost.

For outpatients who are so gravely disabled or who have such impaired judgment that they cannot care for themselves in the community without legally sanctioned supervision, obtaining conservatorship status needs to become easier. For instance, conservatorship in California has become an important therapeutic modality for such persons (Lamb and Weinberger, 1993). The conservator may be granted a number of powers over the mentally ill person. Most commonly granted are powers related to the conservatee's residential placement, his or her involvement in psychiatric treatment, and management of his or her money. The conservator has the authority to place the conservatee in any setting—for example, at home, in a board-and-care facility, or in a psychiatric hospital—and to require that he or she participate in psychiatric treatment and take medications in order to remedy or prevent the recurrence of severe disability.

Conservatorship is particularly effective when conservators are psychiatric social workers or persons with similar backgrounds and skills who use their court-granted authority to become a crucial source of stability and support for chronically mentally ill persons. Conservatorship thus can enable individuals who might otherwise be long-term residents of hospitals to live in the community and achieve a considerable measure of autonomy and satisfaction in their lives.

A system of coordination among funding sources and implementation agencies needs to be established. Because the problems of the chronically and severely mentally ill are addressed by multiple public and private authorities, coordination, so lacking in the deinstitutionalization process, needs to become a primary goal. Turf issues have often hindered cooperation, and different agencies serving the same patients have often worked at cross-purposes. The ultimate objectives must be a true system of care rather than a loose network of services and an ease of communication among different types of agencies (for example, psychiatric, social, vocational, and housing).

Some mentally ill persons, even with high-quality treatment and rehabilitation efforts, remain dangerous or gravely disabled. For the small proportion of the chronically and severely mentally ill who do not respond to current methods of treatment and rehabilitation, ongoing structured twenty-four-hour care needs to be available in long-term settings—hospitals, including state hospitals (Bachrach, 1996), or locked, highly structured community alternatives to them such as California's Institutes for Mental Disease (Lamb, 1997).

Unfortunately, too little knowledge about the needs of severely mentally ill persons has found its way into practice (Talbott, 1985). When present, however, such knowledge has led to a much richer life experience and higher quality of life (Lamb, 1982b).

Families of the Chronically and Severely Mentally Ill

Mental health professionals have learned that the chronically and severely mentally ill and their families need advice. Many mentally ill persons lack the ability to cope with routine stress and need tutelage and specific guidance about what to do in many areas of their lives. For instance, a chronically and severely mentally ill person may find himself or herself in a situation that will, if not resolved, precipitate an exacerbation of acute psychosis. Although what the patient needs to do to extricate himself or herself may be very clear to a mental health professional, the patient may be overwhelmed and immobilized by the seeming complexity of it all. Advice and assistance from mental health professionals are crucial.

Managing major mental illness in a relative at home is an immensely difficult task. Families can, and often do, learn by trial and error over a period of years how to help stabilize a mentally ill relative by encouraging the avoidance of excessive stress, having realistic expectations, setting appropriate limits, understanding the patient's problem in tolerating social stimulation, learning how to react to psychotic symptoms, and encouraging medication compliance. But families learn this at great emotional cost that might have been avoided had they been assisted by knowledgeable professionals. Clearly, families deserve better. If mental health professionals themselves learn how to manage chronically and severely mentally ill persons at home, they can then advise the families and make their lives—and the lives of their mentally ill relatives—immeasurably better (Hatfield, 1994).

Mental health professionals can also use families' abilities to play an important role in the treatment process. To do so, they have to learn to help families set limits and take charge of their households (Kanter, 1985). They have to feel comfortable in telling the family that schizophrenia and other major mental disorders are biological illnesses and that the family has not caused them. They have to be unambivalent about the use of psychoactive medications and in advising families to urge their relatives to take them. They have to work with the families and their mentally ill relatives to determine what are realistic goals. They also need to help relatives understand that social withdrawal may be a necessary defense for mentally ill persons against too much stress or social stimulation, but that excessive withdrawal may lead to a form of institutionalism in the home. A balance must be struck.

A significant development in the last two decades of the twentieth century was the establishment and growth of the National Alliance for the Mentally Ill. This organization was formed by relatives of mentally ill persons and has become not only a very important source of support for family members, but also a major force for advocacy at federal, state, and local levels for chronically and severely mentally ill persons.

Homeless Mentally Ill Persons

Homeless mentally ill persons have become one of the greatest challenges to public mental health, and to society in general. This problem takes on increased importance because of evidence that one-third to one-half of all long-term homeless adults in the United States have a major mental illness (schizophrenia, schizoaffective disorder, bipolar disorder, or major depression) and up to four-fifths have major mental illness or a severe substance use disorder, or both (Baum and Burnes, 1993).

The two American Psychiatric Association task forces on the homeless mentally ill (Lamb, 1984; Lamb, Bachrach, and Kass, 1992) concluded that this problem is the result not of deinstitutionalization itself but of the way it has been implemented. Homelessness among chronically and severely mentally ill persons is symptomatic of the grave problems facing such persons generally in the United States. Thus, the problem of homelessness will not be resolved until these basic underlying problems are addressed and a comprehensive and integrated system of care is established for this population.

The solutions for homelessness among the mentally ill, then, are the same as those enumerated above under "Some Basic Needs of Chronically and Severely Mentally Ill Persons in the Community." Of special importance here is the nation's affordable housing crisis. Many subsidized units of housing for people with disabilities, including people with mental illness, have been lost due to changes in federal housing policy (Consortium for Citizens with Disabilities, 1996).

How do chronically and severely mentally ill individuals become homeless? Obviously, there are many paths to the streets, and a brief look at some of them may be useful. Chronically and severely mentally ill persons are not proficient at coping with the stresses of this world; therefore, they are vulnerable to eviction from their living arrangements, sometimes because of an inability to deal with difficult or even ordinary landlord-tenant situations (Lamb and Talbott, 1986) and sometimes because of circumstances in which they play a leading role. In the absence of an adequate case management system, these individuals are often out on the streets and on their own. Many, especially the young, have a tendency to drift away from their families or from board-and-care homes; they may be trying to escape the pull of dependency and may not be ready to come to terms with living in a sheltered, low-pressure environment. If they still have goals, they may find an inactive lifestyle extremely depressing, or they may want more freedom to drink or use drugs. Some chronically and severely mentally ill persons may regard leaving their comparatively static milieu as a necessary part of the process of realizing their goals, but this process exacts its price in terms of homelessness, crises, decompensation, and hospitalizations.

Once mentally ill persons are out on their own, they more than likely stop taking their medications; after a while, they lose touch with the Social Security Administration and are no longer able to receive their Supplemental Security Income checks. Their poor judgment and the state of disarray associated with their illness may cause them to fail to notify the Social Security Administration of a change of address or to fail to appear for a redetermination hearing. The lack of medical care on the streets and the effects of alcohol and other drug abuse are additional serious complications. These persons may become too disorganized to extricate themselves from living on the streets except by exhibiting blatantly bizarre or disruptive behavior that leads to their being taken to a hospital or jail.

There is still another factor. Evidence is beginning to emerge that homeless mentally ill persons have a greater severity of illness than do mentally ill persons in general. At Bellevue Hospital in New York City, for example, approximately 50 percent of inpatients who are homeless on admission are transferred to state hospitals for long-term care as opposed to 8 percent of other Bellevue psychiatric inpatients (Marcos, Cohen, Nardacci, and Brittain, 1990).

The Mentally Ill in the Criminal Justice System

Since the 1970s, much concern has been expressed about the numbers of mentally ill persons found in U.S. jails and prisons (Swank and Winer, 1976; Stelovich, 1979; Whitmer, 1980; Torrey, 1997). To what extent this is related to deinstitutionalization has been the subject of considerable research (Teplin, 1983, 1990; Davis, 1992). Although some evidence has supported the premise that an increase has taken place, this is difficult to prove because we have no reliable estimates of the numbers of mentally ill persons in jails and prisons prior to deinstitutionalization with which to compare postdeinstitutionalization data. Nevertheless, two factors lead to the general belief that there has indeed been an increase since deinstitutionalization: the very large numbers of mentally ill persons currently residing in jails and prisons and the observations of both clinicians and researchers that a high proportion of mentally ill persons found today in the criminal justice system resemble in most respects the persons who used to be patients in long-term state hospitals.

As a result of deinstitutionalization, large numbers of mentally ill persons now reside in the community. At the same time, community psychiatric resources, including hospital beds, are few. Society has a limited tolerance for mentally disordered behavior, and the result is pressure to institutionalize persons who need twenty-four-hour care wherever there is room, including jail. Indeed, a criminalization of mentally disordered behavior has been described—a shunting of mentally ill persons in need of treatment into the criminal justice system instead of the mental health system (Torrey, 1997; Teplin, 1990). Rather than hospitalization and psychiatric treatment, mentally ill persons who have committed minor crimes often are subject to inappropriate arrest and incarceration. An additional factor in this regard is that many severely mentally ill persons who used to live out their lives in state hospitals are now in the community, where they have the opportunity to come to the attention of the police for what is perceived as criminal behavior. Such behavior is often a manifestation of their illness.

It is important to distinguish major crime from minor crime in determining why a mentally ill person is arrested rather than taken to a hospital. Generally, persons who are thought to have committed a felony are arrested and brought to jail regardless of their mental condition. The criminal justice system, charged by society with removing from the community persons accused of committing serious crimes, sees no alternative but first to place the person in custody in a secure setting and then to arrange for psychiatric treatment, if necessary (Lamb and Grant, 1982).

The situation is different for mentally ill persons who are thought to have committed minor offenses. One can look at this matter from the perspective of what happens in the everyday interaction between the police and the mentally ill or from a more global perspective. Let us examine the former perspective first. A large proportion of acutely mentally ill persons come to the attention of the police (McNiel and others, 1991; Zealberg and others, 1992; Way, Evans, and Banks, 1993; Lamb and others, 1995). Even if psychiatric facilities, both inpatient and outpatient, are available, a detainee's mental illness may not be obvious to police officers, who, despite their practical experience, have not had sufficient training in dealing with this population and are still laypersons in such matters (Husted and Nehemkis, 1995; Husted, Charter, and Perrou, 1995). Moreover, mental illness may appear to the police to be simply alcohol or drug intoxication, especially if the person has been using drugs or alcohol at the time of arrest. Still another factor is that in the heat and confusion of an encounter with the police and other citizens, which may include being forcibly subdued, signs of mental illness can go unnoticed (Lamb and Grant, 1982).

Even if the police do consider the problem to be mental illness, taking the person to a mental hospital can involve problems and aggravation. Among these are long waiting periods in an emergency room, questioning of the judgment of police officers by mental health professionals, and, for mentally ill persons who are admitted, very brief hospital stays for individuals deemed by the police just a short time before to constitute a clear menace to the community (Lamb, Schock, Chen, and Gross, 1984; Rogers, 1990; Laberge and Morin, 1995). On the other hand, if the police book the mentally ill person into jail, they know that he or she will be kept in custody, at least until arraignment, and will perhaps receive psychiatric evaluation and treatment (Jemelka, Trupin, and Chiles, 1989; Laberge and Morin, 1995). In this era of deinstitutionalization, the criminal justice system has taken the place of the state hospitals in becoming the institution that cannot say no (Borzecki and Wormith, 1985).

Other, more global factors are commonly cited as causes of the mentally ill being placed in the criminal justice system. One of them is deinstitutionalization in conjunction with the unavailability of lengthy stays in state hospitals for the chronically and severely mentally ill. The drastically reduced number of state hospital beds lends credence to the validity of this assertion. Other factors mentioned include more formal and more rigid criteria for civil commitment, the lack of adequate support systems for the mentally ill in the community, and the difficulty experienced by mentally ill persons coming from the criminal justice system in gaining access to mental health treatment generally and community treatment appropriate to their particular needs (Teplin, 1996)—for example, outreach services, specialized case management services for this population (Dvoskin and Steadman, 1994), or an agency with the ability to provide the degree of control and structure often required for successful treatment of mentally ill offenders.

A range of effective strategies has been developed to prevent severely mentally ill persons from entering the criminal justice system and, once there, being diverted from it to mental health treatment (Lamb and Weinberger, 1998; Seaman, Barbara, and Dennis, 1994). These include taking steps to prevent the inappropriate arrest of mentally ill persons and providing mental health consultation to police in the field so as to increase the number of mentally ill persons who are given access to the mental health system rather than being jailed (Lamb and others, 1995). Such strategies need widespread and comprehensive implementation.

This subject of the mentally ill in the criminal justice system is discussed in much greater detail in Chapter Three.

The Limits of Deinstitutionalization

In the view of some, deinstitutionalization has gone too far in terms of attempting to treat long-term mentally ill persons in the community. Some long-term mentally ill persons clearly require a highly structured, locked, twenty-four-hour setting for adequate intermediate or long-term management (Dorwart, 1988). The majority of mental health professionals who actually treat patients believe that for those who need such care, society should provide it (Group for the Advancement of Psychiatry, 1982), in either a hospital or an alternative setting such as California's locked Institutes for Mental Disease (Lamb, 1997).

Although community mental health and civil rights movements have made where to treat an ideological issue, such decisions are best based on the clinical needs of each individual. Unfortunately, deinstitutionalization efforts have, in practice, too often confused locus of care and quality of care (Bachrach, 1978). Where mentally ill persons are treated has been seen as more important than how or how well they are treated. Care in the community has often been assumed almost by definition to be better than hospital care. In actuality, poor care can be found in both hospital and community settings. Appropriateness must also be addressed. The long-term mentally ill are not a homogeneous population; what is appropriate for some is inappropriate for others.

The Emergence of Managed Care

The fact that services for chronically and severely mentally ill persons are now out in the community and not systematically managed has created a number of problems in public sector mental health systems. As Hoge and colleagues (1994) have observed, these problems include difficulty finding and accessing services, denial of services to patients who need them, lack of accountability and follow-up for individual patients, absence of coordination among providers, lack of continuity in treatment planning, reimbursement schemes containing disincentives for community-based and rehabilitative treatments, few if any incentives for efficiency or cost saving, and inadequate systems for monitoring the necessity, appropriateness, and effectiveness of care. In an effort to solve these problems, and in particular to make community care more cost-effective, a number of the main elements of managed care have been introduced in such arenas as Medicaid-funded mental health services. Here the potential exists for a significant impact, both positive and negative, on chronically and severely mentally ill persons.

We have already seen how case management has been introduced into public mental health, especially for chronically and severely mentally ill persons, to deal with many of the already noted problems. For instance, case management establishes single-point accountability for the care of individual patients, improves access to services, and promotes continuity of both treatment planning and care. Case management has also been widely employed in the private sector of the health care system as part of managed care to achieve the same goals and to facilitate cost containment. Another important method that has been used to deal with such problems is assertive community treatment, already mentioned.

An in-depth discussion of managed care in the public sector and in Medicaid is beyond the scope here. Capitation will be used to illustrate some of the promise and the pitfalls of the managed care approach. Capitation is an arrangement whereby an agency is given a fixed amount of money to provide all aspects of needed mental health care for a particular group of patients (Mechanic and Aiken, 1989). It has become a cornerstone of managed health care, in both the private and public sectors. Usually the agency is given considerable flexibility as to how these funds are spent as long as the patients' needs are met. In mental health, capitation is most often used to encourage providers to serve the most seriously ill. This funding mechanism is yet another way to establish single-point accountability for care. Moreover, because capitation involves giving an agency a fixed amount of money per patient, it is designed to provide strong incentives for cost efficiency, as well as early treatment and crisis intervention to avert costly psychiatric hospitalization. Capitation should also facilitate coordination, because all services are delivered or purchased by one provider (Lehman, 1987).

Managed care often involves the shifting of responsibility for providing mental health care to a population (for example, the chronically and severely mentally ill) from the public to the private sector. This is based on the belief, backed by recent evidence, that the private sector, unencumbered by the bureaucratic inefficiencies of government, can provide mental health services at a lower cost (Shore, 1996). Even if this is true, a grossly underfunded public system may be equally underfunded when privatized. In addition, capitation, if not closely monitored, can result in undertreatment—or lower-quality treatment—because the agency receives a fixed amount of money per patient regardless of what, or how few or many, services are provided to the patient. Moreover, a managed care approach may reduce or even eliminate patient choice with respect to type of treatment.

Conclusion

Deinstitutionalization is now an accomplished fact. We have taken away from the chronically and severely mentally ill the almost total asylum from the pressures of the world and the care, however imperfect, that they received in state hospitals. The central problem that now needs to be addressed is society's obligation to provide in the community the care and treatment that they need. With the advent of the modern antipsychotic medications and psychosocial treatments, the great majority of such individuals are able to live in a range of open settings in the community: with family, in their own apartments, in board-and-care homes, in halfway houses, and so on. Nevertheless, a minority of persons with chronic and severe mental illness still need highly structured, twenty-four-hour care, often in locked facilities. The fact that a significant proportion of this minority are not receiving such care but are instead living in jails, on the streets, and in other unacceptable situations (Lamb, 1997) is evidence that adequate community care has not been provided for many of the most severely ill. Moreover, we may have deinstitutionalized some mentally ill persons who cannot be effectively treated without highly structured, twenty-four-hour care. But overall, most chronically and severely mentally ill persons now live in the community rather than in institutions. With adequate treatment and support, this change has greatly improved their lot, leading to a much richer life experience and a higher quality of life. We have learned what must be done to bring this about. Now we need the will and the funding to realize the potential of deinstitutionalization to improve the lives of severely mentally ill persons.

References

Andreasen, N. C. "Negative Symptoms in Schizophrenia: Definition and Reliability." *Archives of General Psychiatry,* 1982, *39,* 784–788.

Bachrach, L. L. "A Conceptual Approach to Deinstitutionalization." *Hospital and Community Psychiatry,* 1978, *29,* 573–578.

Bachrach, L. L. "The State of the State Mental Hospital in 1996." *Psychiatric Services,* 1996, *47,* 1071–1078.

Baum, A. S., and Burnes, D. W. (eds.). *A Nation in Denial: The Truth About Homelessness.* Boulder, Colo.: Westview Press, 1993.

Borzecki, M., and Wormith, J. S. "The Criminalization of Psychiatrically Ill People: A Review with a Canadian Perspective." *Psychiatr J Univ Ottawa,* 1985, *10,* 241–247.

Burns, B. J., and Santos, A. B. "Assertive Community Treatment: An Update of Randomized Trials." *Psychiatric Services,* 1995, *46,* 669–675.

Consortium for Citizens with Disabilities. *Opening Doors: Recommendations for a Federal Policy to Address the Housing Needs of People with Disabilities.* Washington, D.C.: Consortium for Citizens with Disabilities, 1996.

Davis, S. "Assessing the 'Criminalization' of the Mentally Ill in Canada." *Canadian Journal of Psychiatry,* 1992, *37,* 532–538.

Dincin, J. (ed.). *A Pragmatic Approach to Psychiatric Rehabilitation: Lessons from Chicago's Thresholds Program.* New Directions for Mental Health Services, no. 68. San Francisco: Jossey-Bass, 1995.

Dorwart, R. A. "A Ten-Year Follow-Up Study of the Effects of Deinstitutionalization." *Hospital and Community Psychiatry,* 1988, *39,* 287–291.

Dvoskin, J. A., and Steadman, H. J. "Using Intensive Case Management to Reduce Violence by Mentally Ill Persons in the Community." *Hospital and Community Psychiatry,* 1994, *45,* 679–684.

Goffman, E. *Asylums: Essays on the Social Situation of Mental Patients and Other Inmates.* New York: Doubleday, 1961.

Group for the Advancement of Psychiatry. *The Positive Aspects of Long-Term Hospitalization in the Public Sector for Chronic Psychiatric Patients.* New York: Mental Health Materials Center, 1982.

Hatfield, A. B. (ed.). *Family Interventions in Mental Illness.* New Directions for Mental Health Services, no. 62. San Francisco: Jossey-Bass, 1994.

Hoffman, B. F. "The Criminalization of the Mentally Ill." *Canadian Journal of Psychiatry,* 1990, *35,* 166–169.

Hoge, M. A., and others. "Defining Managed Care in Public-Sector Psychiatry." *Hospital and Community Psychiatry,* 1994, *45,* 1085–1089.

Hopper, K., Baxter, E., and Cox, S. "Not Making It Crazy: The Young Homeless Patients in New York City." In B. Pepper and H. Ryglewicz (eds.), *The Young Adult Chronic Patient.* New Directions for Mental Health Services, no. 14. San Francisco: Jossey-Bass, 1982.

Husted, J. R., Charter, R. A., and Perrou, B. "California Law Enforcement Agencies and the Mentally Ill Offender." *Bulletin of the American Academy of Psychiatry and Law,* 1995, *23,* 315–329.

Husted, J. R., and Nehemkis, A. "Civil Commitment Viewed from Three Perspectives: Professional, Family, and Police." *Bulletin of the American Academy of Psychiatry and Law,* 1995, *23,* 533–546.

Jemelka, R., Trupin, E., and Chiles, J. A. "The Mentally Ill in Prisons: A Review." *Hospital and Community Psychiatry,* 1989, *40,* 481–491.

Johnstone, E. C., and others. "Institutionalism and the Defects of Schizophrenia." *British Journal of Psychiatry,* 1981, *139,* 195–203.

Kanter, J. S. (ed.). *Clinical Issues in Treating the Chronic Mentally Ill.* New Directions for Mental Health Services, no. 27. San Francisco: Jossey-Bass, 1985.

Laberge, D., and Morin, D. "The Overuse of Criminal Justice Dispositions: Failure of Diversionary Policies in the Management of Mental Health Problems." *International Journal of Law and Psychiatry,* 1995, *18,* 389–414.

Lamb, H. R. "The New Asylums in the Community." *Archives of General Psychiatry,* 1979, *36,* 129–134.

Lamb, H. R. "Young Adult Chronic Patients: The New Drifters." *Hospital and Community Psychiatry,* 1982a, *33,* 465–468.

Lamb, H. R. *Treating the Long-Term Mentally Ill.* San Francisco: Jossey-Bass, 1982b.

Lamb, H. R. (ed.). *The Homeless Mentally Ill: A Task Force Report of the American Psychiatric Association.* Washington, D.C.: American Psychiatric Association, 1984.

Lamb, H. R. "Lessons Learned from Deinstitutionalization in the United States." *British Journal of Psychiatry,* 1993, *162,* 587–592.

Lamb, H. R. "The New State Mental Hospitals in the Community." *Psychiatric Services,* 1997, *48,* 1307–1310.

Lamb, H. R., Bachrach, L. L., and Kass, F. I. (eds.). *Treating the Homeless Mentally Ill: A Report of the Task Force on the Homeless Mentally Ill.* Washington, D.C.: American Psychiatric Association, 1992.

Lamb, H. R., and Grant, R. W. "The Mentally Ill in an Urban County Jail." *Archives of General Psychiatry,* 1982, *39,* 17–22.

Lamb, H. R., and Mills, M. J. "Needed Changes in Law and Procedure for the Chronically Mentally Ill." *Hospital and Community Psychiatry,* 1986, *37,* 475–480.

Lamb, H. R., Schock, R., Chen, P. W., and Gross, B. "Psychiatric Needs in Local Jails: Emergency Issues." *American Journal of Psychiatry,* 1984, *141,* 774–777.

Lamb, H. R., and Talbott, J. A. "The Homeless Mentally Ill: The Perspective of the American Psychiatric Association." *Journal of the American Medical Association,* 1986, *256,* 498–501.

Lamb H. R., and Weinberger, L. E. "Therapeutic Use of Conservatorship in the Treatment of Gravely Disabled Psychiatric Patients." *Hospital and Community Psychiatry,* 1993, *44,* 147–150.

Lamb, H. R., and Weinberger, L. E. "The Mentally Ill in Jails and Prisons: A Review." *Psychiatric Services,* 1998, *49,* 483–492.

Lamb, H. R., and others. "Outcome for Psychiatric Emergency Patients Seen by an Outreach Police–Mental Health Team." *Psychiatric Services,* 1995, *46,* 1267–1271.

Lehman, A. F. "Capitation Payment and Mental Health Care: A Review of Opportunities and Risks." *Hospital and Community Psychiatry,* 1987, *38,* 31–38.

Marcos, L. R., Cohen, N. L., Nardacci, D., and Brittain, J. "Psychiatry Takes to the Streets: The New York City Initiative for the Homeless Mentally Ill." *American Journal of Psychiatry,* 1990, *147,* 1557–1561.

McNiel, D. E., and others. "Characteristics of Persons Referred by Police to the Psychiatric Emergency Room." *Hospital and Community Psychiatry,* 1991, *42,* 425–427.

Mechanic, D., and Aiken, L. H. (eds.). *Paying for Services: Promises and Pitfalls of Capitation.* New Directions for Mental Health Services, no. 43. San Francisco: Jossey-Bass, 1989.

Minkoff, K. "Beyond Deinstitutionalization: A New Ideology for the Postinstitutional Era." *Hospital and Community Psychiatry*, 1987, *38*, 945–950.

Minkoff, K., and Drake, R. E. (eds.). *Dual Diagnosis of Major Mental Illness and Substance Disorder*. New Directions for Mental Health Services, no. 50. San Francisco: Jossey-Bass, 1991.

Mueser, K. T., Douglas, M. S., Bellack, A. S., and Morrison, R. L. "Assessment of Enduring Deficit and Negative Symptom Subtypes in Schizophrenia." *Schizophrenia Bulletin*, 1991, *17*, 565–582.

Pepper, B., Kirshner, M. C., and Ryglewicz, H. "The Young Adult Chronic Patient: Overview of a Population." *Hospital and Community Psychiatry*, 1981, *32*, 463–469.

Rogers, A. "Policing Mental Disorder: Controversies, Myths and Realities." *Soc Policy Admin*, 1990, *24*, 2226–2236.

Seaman, T. J., Barbara, S. S., and Dennis, D. L. "A National Survey of Jail Diversion Programs for Mentally Ill Detainees." *Psychiatric Services*, 1994, *45*, 1109–1113.

Shore, M. F. (ed.). *Managed Care, the Private Sector, and Medicaid Mental Health and Substance Abuse Services*. New Directions for Mental Health Services, no. 72. San Francisco: Jossey-Bass, 1996.

Stein, L. I. "Innovating Against the Current." In L. I. Stein (ed.), *Innovative Community Health Programs*. New Directions for Mental Health Services, no. 56. San Francisco: Jossey-Bass, 1992.

Stelovich, S. "From the Hospital to the Prison: A Step Forward in Deinstitutionalization?" *Hospital and Community Psychiatry*, 1979, *30*, 618–620.

Survey and Analysis Branch, Center for Mental Health Services. *Resident Patients in State and County Mental Hospitals, 1998 Survey*. Washington, D.C.: Substance Abuse and Mental Health Services Administration, U.S. Department of Health and Human Services, 1998.

Swank, G. E., and Winer, D. "Occurrence of Psychiatric Disorder in a County Jail Population." *American Journal of Psychiatry*, 1976, *133*, 1331–1333.

Swanson, J. W., and others. "Interpreting the Effectiveness of Involuntary Outpatient Commitment: A Conceptual Model." *Journal of the American Academy of Psychiatry and Law*, 1997, *25*, 5–16.

Talbott, J. A. "The Fate of the Public Psychiatric System." *Hospital and Community Psychiatry*, 1985, *36*, 46–50.

Talbott, J. A., and Lamb, H. R. "Summary and Recommendations." In H. R. Lamb (ed.), *The Homeless Mentally Ill*. Washington, D.C.: American Psychiatric Association, 1984.

Teplin, L. A. "The Criminalization of the Mentally Ill: Speculation in Search of Data." *Psychological Bulletin*, 1983, *94*, 54–67.

Teplin, L. A. "The Prevalence of Severe Mental Disorder Among Male Urban Jail Detainees: Comparison with the Epidemiologic Catchment Area Program." *American Journal of Public Health*, 1990, *80*, 663–669.

Teplin, L. A. "Prevalence of Psychiatric Disorders Among Incarcerated Women, I: Pretrial Jail Detainees." *Archives of General Psychiatry*, 1996, *53*, 505–512.

Torrey, E. F. *Out of the Shadows: Confronting America's Mental Illness Crisis*. New York: Wiley, 1997.

Van Putten, T., Crumpton, E., and Yale, C. "Drug Refusal in Schizophrenia and the Wish to Be Crazy." *Archives of General Psychiatry*, 1976, *33*, 1443–1446.

Way, B. B., Evans, M. E., and Banks, S. M. "An Analysis of Police Referrals to Ten Psychiatric Emergency Rooms." *Bulletin of the American Academy of Psychiatry and Law*, 1993, *21*, 389–397.

Whitmer, G. E. "From Hospitals to Jails: The Fate of California's Deinstitutionalized Mentally Ill." *American Journal of Orthopsychiatry*, 1980, *50*, 65–75.

Wing, J. K. "The Functions of Asylum." *British Journal of Psychiatry*, 1990, *157*, 822–827.

Wing, J. K., and Brown, G. W. *Institutionalism and Schizophrenia: A Comparative Study of Three Mental Hospitals, 1960–1968*. Cambridge: Cambridge University Press, 1970.

Zealberg, J. J., and others. "A Mobile Crisis Program: Collaboration Between Emergency Psychiatric Services and Police." *Hospital and Community Psychiatry*, 1992, *43*, 612–615.

H. RICHARD LAMB is professor of psychiatry and the behavioral sciences at Keck School of Medicine, University of Southern California, in Los Angeles.

2

*Serious problems result when the community alternatives
to state hospitalization, often driven by lower costs and
an ideology that highly structured care is seldom needed,
are not adequate to meet the needs of those who are
severely mentally ill.*

The New State Mental Hospitals
in the Community

H. Richard Lamb

Between 1955 and 1994 the Untied States reduced its number of occupied
state psychiatric hospital beds from 339 per 100,000 population to 29 per
100,000 on any given day (Resident Patients in State and County Mental
Hospitals, 1994). Some individual states have gone even further. California,
for example, now has four state hospital beds per 100,000 population, not
including forensic patients. Nevertheless, many continue to believe that
state hospitals should be further downsized (Carling, 1995; Okin, 1995;
Becker, 1993; Bachrach, 1996).

Where have all the state hospital patients gone? With the advent of
modern antipsychotic medications and psychosocial treatments, the great
majority are able to live in a range of open settings in the community—with
family, in their own apartments, in board-and-care homes, in halfway
houses, and in similar other settings. Nevertheless, there remains a minority of persons with chronic and severe mental illness who need highly structured, twenty-four-hour care, often in locked facilities (Appleby and others,
1993; Talbott and Glick, 1986). As state hospital beds become scarcer, many
of these mentally ill persons in the various states are housed in correctional
facilities, locked nursing homes, and a variety of other settings (Bachrach,
1996).

In California in the 1970s and 1980s, many medium- or long-term
patients who remained in state hospitals were moved to locked community
facilities with a moderate but lesser degree of structure (Lamb, 1980), now
called institutes for mental disease (IMDs). Similarly, many of the new generation of severely mentally ill persons who grew up since deinstitutionalization were admitted to these facilities. Still, a sizable number of persons

Source: Lamb, H.R. "The New State Mental Hospitals in the Community." *Psychiatric Services*, 1997, *48* (10),
1307–1310. Reprinted by permission.

were judged to need the high degree of structure provided in a state hospital, and this hard-core group remained in the state hospitals.

In the past few years, however, as fiscal shortages have beset state and local mental health authorities, the relatively large per diem costs of state hospitals—in California, approximately $350 a day for long-term patients—have been seen as expenses to cut in order to fund community programs. Since 1993, the county departments of mental health have acted as gatekeepers for, and have paid for the care of, IMD patients from their counties. Thus the IMDs, though privately owned and operated, no longer decide who will be admitted. As a result, throughout California, the tendency has been to transfer patients with increasingly difficult problems in management to IMDs.

The cost to the county departments of mental health for these facilities is $79 a day. This amount is based on the rate for skilled nursing facilities in fiscal year 1996–1997 and includes $5.72 a day for the special psychiatric treatment program.

The purpose of this study is to examine one of these IMDs—which we can call new state hospitals in the community—and the mentally ill persons who now live in them. What are the characteristics of these residents? How has the new trend to treat more and more patients who before 1993 were treated in the state hospitals changed the IMDs? Are these facilities adequate for their new purpose?

Methods

The Study Setting. The facility chosen for this study was a ninety-five-bed locked IMD located in a small city twenty-five miles east of downtown Los Angeles. California currently has forty such facilities, which have a total of approximately four thousand beds. The facility selected is one generally held in high regard by mental health professionals in the area. It is owned and administered by an active member of the National Alliance for the Mentally Ill. The patients come from various counties of southern California. The length of stay averages ten months, an average set by and strongly encouraged by the counties.

The IMD has a pleasant and attractive physical appearance. It was built in 1970 as a skilled nursing facility for geriatric patients and was converted to its present use in 1971, primarily by locking the doors, bolting the windows shut, and substituting transparent plastic windows for regular glass windows.

The facility provides very close medication supervision, with approximately three-fifths of the patients receiving their medication in either liquid or crushed form. The staff-patient ratio is high; the facility has forty-five full-time nursing staff members, eighteen of whom are licensed (registered nurses, licensed practical nurses, or psychiatric technicians). The staff includes three part-time psychiatrists, each of whom spends about two and a half to three hours a week at the facility.

Staffing also includes fourteen program staff members who have bachelor's degrees and prior experience with psychiatric patients and who provide at least twenty-seven hours of activities a week for each patient. Activities include group therapies, therapeutic social and recreational activities, and instruction in activities of daily living such as using public transportation. Three adult education teachers paid by the local school district spend half to three-quarters of their time in the facility.

Procedure. During the study, I served as a volunteer staff psychiatrist at the facility. One hundred one patients who had been at the facility for at least a month were randomly selected as study subjects. The study data were obtained from the medical records and from discussion of each case with the staff. Data collection took place from January through June 1996.

Results

Fifty-nine of the subjects were men, and forty-two were women. The median age of the sample was thirty-eight years, with a range of eighteen to fifty-four years, and the median age for men and for women was also thirty-eight. Sixty-one of the subjects were white, twenty-one were black, fifteen were Hispanic, three were Pacific Islanders, and one was Asian.

Of the 101 subjects, 68 (67 percent) had a diagnosis of schizophrenia, 26 (26 percent) of schizoaffective disorder, six (6 percent) of bipolar disorder, and one (1 percent) of dementia due to head trauma. Ninety-nine (98 percent) were under psychiatric conservatorship on admission and thus were signed in by their conservators. Two (2 percent) were voluntary admissions.

All of the sample had prior psychiatric hospitalizations. Thirteen (13 percent) had been long-term state hospital patients with stays of two to fifteen years. Seventy-seven (76 percent) had a history of serious physical violence against persons, and 71 (70 percent) were known to have had problems with substance abuse.

Ninety-seven patients (96 percent) had a history of poor medication compliance. In the facility, psychotropic medications were prescribed for all the study patients, though in one case, the patient's knowledge of martial arts prevented the staff from administering them. Ninety-four patients (93 percent) continued to exhibit psychotic symptoms after admission, even while on medications. Forty-four (44 percent) had been violent toward persons during the current admission. Statistical analysis showed a relationship between violence during the current admission and history of physical violence against persons ($\chi^2 = 17.81$, df = 1, $p < .001$, corrected for continuity).

Four patients were known to be firesetters, and four tended to make repeated inappropriate 911 calls. Many patients displayed unacceptable sexual behavior, such as exhibiting themselves or masturbating in public; others tended to urinate or defecate in public places.

As a result of patient violence, the study facility averages two staff injuries and more than four patient injuries a month that require medical attention. Before 1993, such injuries were very infrequent, and the total was not tabulated. During the study period, one staff member was on disability leave for two weeks as a result of head trauma. Records are not kept for slaps, pinches, hair pulling, sexual grabbing, and similar incidents that do not require first aid.

Discussion

The population studied presented extremely difficult problems in management and treatment. A large percentage of patients were characterized by a history of serious violence against persons, psychotic diagnoses, current presence of psychosis despite antipsychotic medications, a history of poor compliance with psychotropic medications, lack of internal controls, and problems with substance abuse when not in a structured setting. These factors are some of the most important predictors of dangerousness for severely mentally ill persons (Mulvey, 1994). The relationship found in this study between violence in the facility and a history of violence is consistent with previous findings on the relationship between current and past violence.

Thirteen percent of the study population had been long-stay state hospital patients (two years or more of hospitalization) before coming to the IMD, and probably many others came to the facility as an alternative to becoming long-stay state hospital patients. By simply walking through the units, one could see bizarre behavior exhibited by many patients; the "chronic" look of many patients despite an active and high-quality rehabilitation program; and staff's increasing fearfulness of what they described as the ever-present threat of violence, a phenomenon new to this facility. Moreover, patients frequently kicked holes in the walls and otherwise caused costly damage to the facility, which was not built to withstand physical violence.

In the past, this facility had treated mentally ill persons who were judged to need a locked, structured setting but not the high degree of security, physical structure, and control provided in a state hospital (Lamb, 1980). The facility had provided much of that structure through the intensive treatment and rehabilitation program. Patients who were felt to need the higher degree of structure found in state hospitals were not accepted here. Now the facility has the atmosphere and feel of a state hospital with a hard-core population of mentally ill persons who present difficult problems in management that cannot be dealt with elsewhere.

It is not surprising that assaultiveness is a problem for some in view of the growing body of evidence that mental illness and violence are related, especially among persons who are psychotic and do not take their medications (Mulvey, 1994; Junginger, 1996; Link and Stueve, 1995; Torrey, 1994; Monahan, 1992). Increasing attention has been paid to staff injuries in psychiatric hospitals (Carmel and Hunter, 1993; Dubin and Lion, 1992; Lion and Reid, 1983). Carmel and Hunter (1993) have observed that violence to staff "affects the atmosphere, programs, staff, and patients of hospitals caring for the mentally ill. It may be difficult to conduct therapeutic programs or retain effective staff in an environment colored by violence by patients" (p. 485). In the IMD studied, injuries to staff and patients occur even though a course for staff on the management of assaultive behavior is given twice a year and the facility tends to hire more and more physically strong male staff.

Ninety-eight percent of the sample were on mental health conservatorship on admission. In California, the court places only the most difficult and consistently treatment-resistant mentally ill persons on conservatorship (Lamb and Weinberger, 1992).

Clearly, there has been a major change in mental health policy in the way that chronically and severely mentally ill persons who present serious problems in management are being treated. At their current rate of reimbursement, IMDs cannot provide a high degree of security and control of violence and a physical plant that can withstand physical violence. Yet that is what many of the patients now being sent to these facilities need. Moreover, the change in locus of care and markedly less structure for the group have come about with little public debate; generally, not only the citizenry but even most mental health professionals are unaware that this change has taken place.

The motivation for this change is not difficult to fathom. It has been shown that shifting responsibility for payment for state hospitals beds from the state to community mental health agencies results in state hospital downsizing (Cuffel, Wait, and Head, 1994). In California, the responsibility for paying for state hospital patient-days has been shifted to the counties, which are in continuous fiscal crisis. Because a state hospital bed day costs approximately $350, compared with $79 for an IMD bed day, the temptation to transfer patients from state hospitals to IMDs is great. Moreover, many people believe, on ideological grounds, that it is important to move as many patients as possible from state hospitals to facilities in the community.

Conclusion

The dramatic reduction in state hospital populations has not been without consequences. Although most chronically and severely mentally ill persons who used to live in state hospitals have adjusted well to living in the community, some continue to need a high degree of structured twenty-four-hour care. The remaining state hospital patients have come to constitute a concentrated hard-core group with especially difficult problems in management, including serious violence against persons, poor compliance with psychotropic medications, and severe problems with substance abuse.

The facility studied here has only a moderate degree of structure. Nevertheless, increasingly difficult and violent patients have been transferred to it in the past several years. The result has been a rising tide of violence, with resulting staff and patient injuries and damage to the facility itself. Both patients and staff now find themselves in a situation that is becoming more and more dangerous and in which treatment and rehabilitation are increasingly difficult to accomplish. There are anecdotal reports that this situation prevails in IMDs throughout the state.

Transfer of patients to community alternatives is too often driven by lower costs and an ideology that highly structured care is seldom needed and that the funding should be used instead for community treatment. On the other hand, more and more persons are advocating that we should first focus on individuals' needs and then create the structures necessary for meeting those needs (Geller and Fisher, 1993; Munetz and Geller, 1993).

This study reflects the violence and the difficulty of providing treatment and rehabilitation that occur when mentally ill persons who have shown a need for a high degree of structure are inappropriately transferred to a lesser level of care that is not equipped to provide that degree of structure. Once again, the most seriously mentally ill are being underserved.

References

Appleby, L., and others. "Length of Stay and Recidivism in Schizophrenia: A Study of Public Psychiatric Hospital Patients." *American Journal of Psychiatry*, 1993, *150*, 72–76.

Bachrach, L. L. "The State of the State Mental Hospital in 1996." *Psychiatric Services*, 1996, *47*, 1071–1078.

Becker, F. W. "The Politics of Closing State Mental Hospitals: A Case of Increasing Policy Gridlock." *Community Mental Health Journal*, 1993, *29*, 103–117.

Carling, P. J. *Return to the Community*. New York: Guilford Press, 1995.

Carmel, H., and Hunter, M. "Staff Injuries from Patient Attack: Five Years' Data." *Bulletin of the American Academy of Psychiatry and the Law*, 1993, *21*, 485–493.

Cuffel, B. J., Wait, D., and Head, T. "Shifting the Responsibility for Payment for State Hospital Services to Community Mental Health Agencies." *Hospital and Community Psychiatry*, 1994, *45*, 460–465.

Dubin, W. R., and Lion, J. R. (eds.). *Clinician Safety: Report of the American Psychiatric Association Task Force on Clinician Safety*. Washington, D.C.: American Psychiatric Association, 1992.

Geller, J. L., and Fisher, W. H. "The Linear Continuum of Transitional Residences: Debunking the Myth." *American Journal of Psychiatry*, 1993, *150*, 1070–1076.

Junginger, J. "Psychosis and Violence: The Case for a Content Analysis of Psychotic Experience." *Schizophrenia Bulletin*, 1996, *22*, 91–103.

Lamb, H. R. "Structure: The Neglected Ingredient of Community Treatment." *Archives of General Psychiatry*, 1980, *37*, 1224–1228.

Lamb, H. R., and Weinberger, L. E. "Conservatorship for Gravely Disabled Psychiatric Patients: A Four-Year Follow-Up Study." *American Journal of Psychiatry*, 1992, *149*, 909–913.

Link, B. G., and Stueve, A. "Evidence Bearing on Mental Illness as a Possible Cause of Violent Behavior." *Epidemiologic Reviews*, 1995, *17*, 172–181.

Lion, J. R., and Reid, W. H. (eds.). *Assaults Within Psychiatric Facilities*. New York: Grune & Stratton, 1983.

Monahan, J. "Mental Disorder and Violent Behavior." *American Psychologist*, 1992, *47*, 511–521.

Mulvey, E. P. "Assessing the Evidence of a Link Between Mental Illness and Violence." *Hospital and Community Psychiatry*, 1994, *45*, 663–668.

Munetz, M. R., and Geller, J. L. "The Least Restrictive Alternative in the Postinstitutional Era." *Hospital and Community Psychiatry*, 1993, *44*, 967–973.

Okin, R. L. "Testing the Limits of Deinstitutionalization." *Psychiatric Services*, 1995, *46*, 569–574.

Resident Patients in State and County Mental Hospitals. *1994 Survey*. Rockville, Md.: Center for Mental Health Services, Survey and Analysis Branch, 1994.

Talbott, J. A., and Glick, I. D. "The Inpatient Care of the Chronically Mentally Ill." *Schizophrenia Bulletin*, 1986, *12*, 129–140.

Torrey, E. F. "Violent Behavior by Individuals with Serious Mental Illness." *Hospital and Community Psychiatry*, 1994, *45*, 653–662.

H. RICHARD LAMB is professor of psychiatry and the behavioral sciences at Keck School of Medicine, University of Southern California, in Los Angeles.

3

One of the greatest problems of deinstitutionalization has been the very large number of persons with severe mental illness who have entered the criminal justice system instead of the mental health system.

Persons with Severe Mental Illness in Jails and Prisons: A Review

H. Richard Lamb, Linda E. Weinberger

Mental health professionals have become increasingly concerned about the number of persons with mental illness in jails and prisons. This issue is a relatively recent one. Reports of large numbers of mentally ill persons in American jails and prisons began appearing in the 1970s (Swank and Winer, 1976; Stelovich, 1979; Whitmer, 1980). This phenomenon had not been reported since the nineteenth century (Torrey, 1997).

To understand this problem better, a literature review was conducted. Two of the primary questions addressed were whether large numbers of persons with severe mental illness who commit legal transgressions are being taken to jails and sent to prisons instead of to hospitals or other psychiatric treatment facilities and whether the number has increased since deinstitutionalization.

The review also examined other aspects of this issue, including the characteristics of mentally ill offenders, factors cited as causes of mentally ill persons' being placed in the criminal justice system, the relationship between mental illness and violence, access to treatment for this population, the role of the police, and society's attitudes toward mentally ill offenders. Finally, recommendations are made about how inappropriate placement of this population in the criminal justice system can be prevented and how to treat mentally ill offenders both in the system and after they are released into the community.

Methods

MEDLINE, *Psychological Abstracts,* and the *Index to Legal Periodicals and Books* were searched from 1970, and all relevant references were obtained.

Source: Lamb, H. R., and Weinberger, L. E. "Persons with Sever Mental Illness in Jails and Prisons: A Review." *Psychiatric Services,* 1998, *49* (4), 483–492. Reprinted by permission.

Results and Discussion

Incarceration Versus Hospitalization. Many factors come into play in determining why a person with mental illness is arrested rather than taken to a hospital. Generally, persons who are thought to have committed a felony are arrested and brought to jail regardless of their mental condition. The criminal justice system, charged by society with the responsibility for removing from the community persons accused of committing serious crimes, sees no alternative but to place the person in custody in a secure setting first and then arrange for psychiatric treatment if necessary (Lamb and Grant, 1982). If the person is thought to have committed a serious crime, the police and the criminal justice system generally do not want to leave this person in a psychiatric hospital where security may be lax, the offense may be seen by staff as secondary to the patient's illness, and the person may be released to the community in a relatively short time.

For persons charged with misdemeanors, the situation becomes more complex. Abramson (1972) was the first to coin the term *criminalization of the mentally ill;* he observed that persons with mental disorders who engaged in minor crimes were increasingly subject to arrest and prosecution in a county jail system. Subsequently, many authors applied the concept of criminalization to persons with mental disorders who were arrested for serious crimes.

The distinction between arrest and incarceration of mentally ill persons who have committed minor offenses and those who have committed serious offenses is an important one. As Steury (1991) notes, no consensus exists on the definition of criminalization of persons with mental disorders. Some researchers define criminalization at the point of arrest (Cocozza, Steadman, and Melick, 1978; Steadman, Cocozza, and Melick, 1978; Schuerman and Kobrin, 1984; Teplin, 1984) and others require prosecution (Dickey, 1980; Hochstedler, 1986, 1987; Arvanites, 1988), while others use incarceration in jails and prisons (Steadman, Vanderwyst, and Ribner, 1978; Teplin, 1983).

In our opinion, the term *criminalization* should be used primarily in connection with mentally ill persons who are arrested with or without jail detention and prosecuted for minor offenses instead of being placed in the mental health system. As noted, it is clear that persons who have committed serious offenses, no matter how mentally ill, would normally be processed in the criminal justice system (Hochstedler, 1986; American Bar Association, 1986; Ogloff and others, 1990). However, it should be acknowledged that many mentally ill persons who commit serious crimes and enter the criminal justice system might not have engaged in such behavior if they had been receiving adequate and appropriate mental health treatment (Dvoskin and Steadman, 1994).

Penrose (1939) advanced the thesis that a relatively stable number of persons are confined in any industrial society. Using prison and mental hospital census data from eighteen European countries, Penrose found an inverse relationship between prison and mental hospital populations. He theorized that if one of these forms of confinement is reduced, the other will increase. According to this theory, where prison populations are extensive, mental hospital populations will be small, and vice versa. Thus, if there is room in prisons and a shortage of hospital beds, many mentally ill persons who come to the attention of law enforcement might well be directed to the criminal justice system. Another corollary of this theory is that if civil commitment is reduced, involvement with the criminal courts will increase (Stone, 1978).

Proportion of Incarcerated Persons with Mental Illness. The Bolton study (Arthur Bolton Associates, 1976) was one of the first extensive and methodologically sound attempts to determine the percentage of county jail inmates with mental illness. In a five-county combined sample of 1,084 adults in California county jails, 6.7 percent were psychotic, and 9.3 percent were judged to have nonpsychotic mental disorders, not including personality disorders. For Los Angeles County, the figures were 7.8 percent psychotic and 5.7 percent nonpsychotic.

In a more recent systematic study, Teplin (1990) interviewed 728 randomly selected male admissions to the Cook County jail in Chicago. Using a structured psychiatric interview, they found that 6.4 percent met diagnostic criteria for schizophrenia, mania, or major depression. In a second study of women entering a county jail in Chicago, Teplin, Abram, and McClelland (1996) found that 15 percent had severe psychiatric disorders within the previous six months, 1.8 percent had schizophrenia or a schizophreniform disorder, 2.2 percent were manic, and 13.7 percent had major depression. Guy and others (1985) interviewed ninety-six randomly selected admissions to the Philadelphia city jail and found that 14.6 percent had schizophrenia or manic-depressive illness.

With regard to state prisons, in a 1987 Michigan study of 1,070 state prison inmates carefully selected through a stratified random sampling procedure, 2.8 percent were found to have schizophrenia, 5.1 percent to have major depression, and 3.8 percent to have bipolar disorder or mania (Neighbors, 1987). Jemelka and others (1992) used the Diagnostic Interview Schedule with 109 inmates in the state of Washington and found prevalence rates of 4.4 percent for schizophrenia, 10.0 percent for major depression, and 3.7 percent for mania. Similar rates were found in California and Ohio prisons (Jemelka, Rahman, and Trupin, 1993). Steadman and others (1987) studied a random sample of 3,332 inmates representing 9.4 percent of New York's general prison population, as well as 352 of the 360 inmates in the prisons' mental health units. They found that 8 percent of the sample had severe psychiatric functional disabilities that clearly warranted some type of mental health intervention, and another 16 percent had significant mental disabilities that required periodic services (specific diagnoses were not given).

Generally, clinical studies suggest that 10 to 15 percent of persons in state prisons have severe mental illness (Jemelka, Rahman, and Trupin, 1993). It may be that in recent years, correctional staff have become better able to recognize signs of mental disturbance and, as a result, refer more of these individuals to mental health professionals. Thus, better recognition may also contribute to the prevalence rate of inmates identified as mentally ill.

The magnitude of the problem can be seen when we multiply the percentages of mentally ill persons in jails and prisons by the number of inmates. For instance, in 1995, there were more than 483,000 persons in jails and more than 1,587,000 persons in state and federal prisons (U.S. Department of Justice, 1995). Thus, even a small percentage of such large populations represents a very significant number of mentally ill persons in jails and prisons.

The large number of mentally ill individuals in jails and prisons has presented serious problems for correctional staff. Gibbs (1983) noted that second to overcrowding, the presence of inmates with psychological problems was the most serious concern for correctional personnel.

Description of the Population. In a study of 102 male inmates of a county jail randomly selected from those referred by jail staff for psychiatric evaluation, 99 percent had previous psychiatric hospitalizations, and 92 percent had arrest records (75 percent for felonies) (Lamb and Grant, 1982). Four-fifths exhibited severe and overt psychopathology, and more than three-fourths met criteria for civil commitment. When arrested, more than a third were transients, and only 12 percent were employed. More than half were currently charged with felonies and 39 percent with crimes of violence. Thus, this population is characterized by extensive experience with both the criminal justice system and the mental health system; severe, acute, and chronic mental illness; and poor functioning.

The same study also found that of those charged with misdemeanors, more than half had been living on the streets, on the beach, in missions, or in cheap hotels, compared with less than a fourth of those charged with felonies (Lamb and Grant, 1982). Persons living in such places obviously have a minimum of community supports. The authors speculated that the less serious misdemeanor offense is frequently a way of asking for help. Still another factor may be that many uncared-for mentally ill persons may be arrested for minor criminal acts that are really manifestations of their illness, their lack of treatment, and the lack of structure in their lives. It was also observed that some inmates, even though overtly psychotic, had underlying antisocial personality problems that appeared to play a major role as causative factors in their alleged criminal behavior. Findings were comparable in a similarly selected sample of 101 inmates of a county jail for women (Lamb and Grant, 1983).

Other studies have shown that a large proportion of mentally ill persons in a jail population were homeless before arrest and incarceration (Michaels and others, 1992; Martell, Rosner, and Harmon, 1995). For instance, one study in New York City found that homeless mentally ill persons were grossly overrepresented among defendants with mental disorders entering the criminal justice and forensic mental health systems for both violent and nonviolent offenses (Martell, Rosner, and Harmon, 1995). Forty-three percent of the defendants with mental disorders were homeless at the time of the crime for which they were arrested. The rate of homelessness was twenty-one times higher in the overall sample of defendants with mental disorders than in the overall population of mentally ill persons in the city. Moreover, homeless defendants were significantly more likely to have been charged with victimizing strangers.

Current Trends. It is often asserted that the number of mentally ill persons currently in our criminal justice system is larger than before deinstitutionalization (Torrey, 1997; Palermo, Smith, and Liska, 1991; Davis, 1992). This assertion is consistent with Penrose's theory described above. It can be argued that society's tolerance in the community of the deviant behavior of people with mental disorders appears to be limited. This limited tolerance is especially true for those who have direct contact with mentally ill persons: the courts, families, and other citizens. Many believe that if social control through the mental health system is impeded because of constraints such as fewer long-term state hospital beds, community pressure will result in placement of some of these persons in the criminal justice system.

In the 1970s, studies began to appear showing that the arrest rate for former psychiatric hospital patients was higher than that for the general population (Zitrin and others, 1976; Sosowsky, 1978). Various attempts were made to account for the higher rate. Steadman, Cocozza, and Melick (1978) concluded from their data that the increase was due almost entirely to the increased number of persons with arrest records being admitted to mental hospitals. They speculated that "persons who formerly would have been caught in the 'revolving cell door' are now bouncing back and forth between state hospitals and jails as solutions are sought in mental health treatment for what are usually nuisance behaviors or property offenses" (p. 820).

A related explanation in the late 1970s was the theory of the "psychiatricization" of criminals (Cocozza, Steadman, and Melick, 1978; Davis, 1992). This theory hypothesized that the increased rate of violent crime after hospital discharge was due to jail and prison overcrowding and that mental hospitals were increasingly admitting individuals formerly dealt with by the criminal justice system. On the other hand, a 1978 study in a California county showed that former hospital patients with no history of arrests when they entered the hospital were arrested roughly three times more often after discharge than the general county population and five times more often for serious violent crimes (Sosowsky, 1980).

Another explanation for the increased arrest rate of former hospital patients is that a more criminal group of mentally ill individuals is now hospitalized as a result of the stricter criteria for civil commitment, which rely heavily on dangerousness (Steadman and others, 1984). Finally, the relationship between mental illness and violence, as discussed below, may be another factor. Despite the arguments offered, sufficient evidence does not exist to settle these issues definitively.

An important question is whether the number of mentally ill persons in jails and prisons has increased since deinstitutionalization. A number of studies over the past several decades have purported to demonstrate an increase, but Teplin (1983) perhaps said it best when she wrote, "It is concluded that the research literature, albeit methodologically flawed, offers at least modest support for the contention that the mentally ill are being [increasingly] processed through the criminal justice system" (p. 54). This evidence is largely clinical and inferential, and it is certainly highly suggestive. However, because of the lack of good studies of mentally ill persons in jails and prisons before deinstitutionalization, findings of research conducted since that time cannot be considered conclusive evidence that the number of mentally ill persons has increased.

Nevertheless, it appears that a greater proportion of mentally ill persons are arrested compared with the general population. One of the better studies suggesting this disproportionate rate was conducted by Teplin (1984). Chicago policemen were observed over a 2,200-hour, fourteen-month period, and 1,382 police-citizen encounters were documented. The presence of psychiatric illness in a suspect was determined at the scene by a system that took into account behavioral symptoms and the environmental context. It was found that 27.9 percent of the suspects without mental disorders and 46.7 percent of the psychiatrically ill suspects were arrested.

Perhaps two of the more persuasive arguments that a higher proportion of persons with severe mental illness can be found in the criminal justice system since deinstitutionalization are the presence of large numbers of such persons now residing in our jails and prisons and the clinical observations of clinicians and researchers. It is the impression of clinicians and researchers that a large proportion of the severely mentally ill persons they see in jails and prisons are similar in almost every way to long-term patients in state hospitals before deinstitutionalization (Lamb, 1982). Obviously, lifetime residents of state hospitals had little opportunity to commit crimes and to be arrested.

In a similar vein, it was observed even in the 1970s that more liberty for the traditional psychiatric hospital patient placed in the community, including the ability to refuse treatment, is likely an important factor in explaining the observed increased arrest rate and violence (Sosowsky, 1978; Grunberg, Klinger, and Grument, 1977). As discussed below, it is generally the untreated mentally ill person who is more violent, particularly if substance abuse is involved.

Mental Illness and Violence. Until recently, it was generally believed that persons with major mental illness such as schizophrenia and bipolar illness were not more likely to commit violent crimes than the general population (Stone, 1997). However, a growing body of evidence has shown a relationship between mental illness and violence, especially among persons who are psychotic and do not take their medications (Monahan, 1992; Torrey, 1994; Mulvey, 1994; Link and Stueve, 1995; Mednick, Brennan, and Katila, 1996; Junginger, 1996; Hodgins and others, 1996; Marzuk, 1996; Swanson and others, 1997b). This relationship is most striking in relatively nonviolent societies, such as in Scandinavia. For instance, Mednick, Brennan, and Katila (1996) found that males in Denmark with a severe mental disorder who were admitted to a psychiatric hospital by age forty-four represented only 5 percent of the total population of males but were responsible for about 30 percent of all the violent offenses committed by males. Similarly, female mental patients in Denmark constituted about 5 percent of the female population but were responsible for 50 percent of all the violent offenses committed by females. Similar findings were noted in Sweden (Hodgins, 1992).

Substance abuse also increases the risk of violent behavior, particularly in combination with severe mental illness (Stone, 1997; Mulvey, 1994; Hodgins and others, 1996; Swanson and others, 1997b; Hodgins, 1992; Steadman, 1997; Fulwiler and others, 1997). Although it would appear that the vast majority of persons with serious mental illness are not more dangerous than the general population, the recent literature cited above suggests the existence of a subgroup that is more dangerous. It has been asserted that violent behavior by this subgroup stigmatizes mentally ill persons generally and that it will be difficult to reduce the stigma until the violence of this subgroup is addressed (Torrey, 1997).

Causative Factors. The factors most commonly cited as causes of mentally ill persons' being placed in the criminal justice system are deinstitutionalization and the unavailability of long-term hospitalization in state hospitals for persons with chronic and severe mental illness, more formal and rigid criteria for civil commitment, the lack of adequate support systems for mentally ill persons in the community, the difficulty mentally ill persons coming from the criminal justice system have gaining access to mental health treatment in the community, and a belief by law enforcement personnel that they can deal with deviant behavior more quickly and efficiently within the criminal justice system than in the mental health system (Laberge and Morin, 1995; Jemelka, Trupin, and Chiles, 1989). A factor less commonly discussed is the public's attitudes toward persons with mental disorders who commit crimes.

In an article about the homeless mentally ill population, Belcher (1988) wrote that "a combination of severe mental illness, a tendency to decompensate in a nonstructured environment, and an inability or unwillingness to follow through with voluntary aftercare arrangements and take prescribed medication contributed to involvement with the criminal justice system. Wandering aimlessly in the community, psychotic much of the time, and unable to manage their internal control systems, these people found the criminal justice system was an asylum of last resort" (p. 193).

Deinstitutionalization. As noted, the belief that deinstitutionalization is a cause of mentally ill persons' being placed in the criminal justice system is a widely held theory for which some evidence exists (Lamb and Grant, 1982; Teplin, 1983). It can certainly be demonstrated that less room currently exists in state mental hospitals for chronically and severely mentally ill persons. In 1955, when the number of patients in state hospitals in the United States reached its highest point, 559,000 persons were institutionalized in state mental hospitals out of a total national population of 165 million. Now the figure is 57,151 for a population of more than 275 million. In about forty years, the United States has reduced its number of occupied state hospital beds from 339 per 100,000 population to 21 per 100,000 on any given day (Survey and Analysis Branch, Center for Mental Health Services, 2000). However, these figures may not accurately reflect the numbers of persons who receive highly structured twenty-four-hour care because of the development and growth of a variety of community psychiatric facilities (many of them locked) in the various states that attempt to provide this kind of care (Lamb, 1997).

In our opinion, deinstitutionalization set the stage for increasing numbers of mentally ill persons to enter the criminal justice system. Moreover, serious problems in implementing deinstitutionalization have often been encountered, such as inadequate or inappropriate outpatient treatment, insufficient community resources, and insufficient twenty-four-hour highly structured psychiatric care facilities for those who need them. To the extent that deinstitutionalization has resulted in these problems, we believe that it is a significant factor accounting for the placement in jails and prisons of many mentally ill persons who would otherwise be treated in the community or in a hospital.

More Restrictive Civil Commitment Criteria. Many people believe that more stringent civil commitment criteria have contributed not only to deinstitutionalization but to an increased number of mentally ill persons in jails and prisons (Laberge and Morin, 1995; Belcher, 1988; Borzecki and Wormith, 1985; Husted and Nehemkis, 1995). In 1969, California's then-novel civil commitment law, the Lanterman-Petris-Short Act, went into effect. Within a decade, every state and Puerto Rico made similar modifications in their commitment codes. Such a rapid and complete consensus among legislatures is virtually unprecedented. More important, it reflected a nearly universal view that past inattention to the rights of mentally ill persons needed to be corrected.

In effect, the new civil commitment laws accomplished three things. First, the laws changed the substantive criteria for commitment from more general criteria that simply embodied concepts of mental illness and need for treatment to more specific criteria that embodied either dangerousness resulting from mental illness or the incapacity to care for oneself. Second, the laws changed the duration of commitment from indeterminate and extensive periods to determinate and brief periods. Third, the new laws explicitly provided that persons civilly committed have rapid access to the courts, attorneys, and, in some cases, jury trials; this access ensured the kinds of due process guarantees to civilly committed persons that criminal defendants had obtained over the previous decade (Lamb and Mills, 1986).

These procedural safeguards and clear commitment standards resulted in fewer as well as shorter commitments. Thus, many mentally ill individuals who would otherwise have been civilly committed by family or others were now left to reside in the community. Moreover, the civil commitment standard for dangerousness in some states, such as Alaska (Alaska, sec. 47.30.740), California (California Welfare and Institutions Code, sec. 5300), and Washington (Revised Code of Washington Annotated [West], sec. 71.05.280), becomes more restrictive when extended commitments are sought. Therefore, only the most dangerous mentally ill persons remain hospitalized, and the less dangerous are discharged. The result is greatly increased numbers of mentally ill persons in the community who may commit criminal acts and enter the criminal justice system.

On the other hand, it has been observed that changes in civil commitment law have often not had in practice the impact intended by those who wrote them (Appelbaum, 1997). These reforms have been resisted by judges, mental health professionals, families, and even attorneys when they were seen as shifting the focus away from patients' treatment needs. Thus, in some instances, more restrictive commitment laws may not have been an important cause of an increased number of mentally ill persons in jail.

Access to Treatment. The availability, or lack of availability, of treatment resources in the community has three important aspects. First, it is clear that in most, though by no means all, jurisdictions in this country, mental health treatment, housing, and rehabilitation resources are insufficient to serve the very large numbers of mentally ill persons in the community (Lamb, 1999). For instance, case management has come to be viewed as one of the essential components of an adequate mental health program (Dvoskin and Steadman, 1994; Steadman and others, 1984; Kanter, 1995). However, the criminal justice system is ill prepared to provide case management services to mentally ill persons who are leaving jails and prisons. In many jurisdictions, local mental health agencies have also been slow to provide these services to this population (Jemelka, Trupin, and Chiles, 1989).

Second, community mental health resources may be inappropriate for the population to be served (Teplin, Abram, and McClelland, 1996). For instance, mentally ill persons may be expected to come to outpatient clinics when the real need for a large proportion of this population is outreach services. Some service providers may lack the ability to provide the degree of structure required by many mentally ill offenders.

Third, mentally ill persons who have been in jail may not be able to gain access to community treatment even when it is available. These persons

have been described as resistant to treatment, dangerous, seriously substance abusing, and "sociopathic" (Jemelka, Trupin, and Chiles, 1989;
Borzecki and Wormith, 1985; Draine, Solomon, and Meyerson, 1994), characteristics generally not considered desirable by most community mental
health agencies. Furthermore, because many of these agencies may not have
the capability to provide the needed structure, limit setting, and safety for
staff necessary to treat these persons successfully, their reluctance to treat
them may be appropriate.

A large proportion of mentally ill persons who commit criminal
offenses tends to be highly resistant to psychiatric treatment (Laberge and
Morin, 1995; Borzecki and Wormith, 1985; Lamb, 1987). They may refuse
referral, may not keep appointments, may not be compliant with psychoactive medications, may not abstain from substance abuse, and may refuse
appropriate housing placements. As Whitmer (1980) has observed, attempts
at outpatient treatment with such persons "take on the aspect of a contest
that a woefully unprepared therapist must sooner or later forfeit" (p. 67).
Hence, he used the term *forfeited patients* to emphasize that these persons
are not just passively lost to treatment, but that mental health professionals
have actively struggled to treat them and have had to acknowledge defeat.

Thus, the mental health system finds these mentally ill offenders
extremely difficult to treat and resists serving them (Laberge and Morin,
1995; Draine, Solomon, and Meyerson, 1994). This reluctance extends to
virtually all areas of community-based care, including therapeutic housing,
social and vocational rehabilitation, and general social services (Jemelka,
Trupin, and Chiles, 1989). Moreover, many mentally ill offenders are intimidating because of previous violent and fear-inspiring behavior. Treating this
group is very different from helping passive, formerly institutionalized
patients adapt quietly to life in the community (Bachrach, Talbott, and Meyerson, 1987). Community mental health professionals are not only reluctant but may also be afraid to treat them, especially when measures are not
adopted to ensure staff safety. Then these mentally ill persons are left for the
criminal justice system to manage (Draine, Solomon, and Meyerson, 1994).
We should add that we have also seen outpatient facilities in which structure is provided, staff are protected, and mental health and criminal justice
staff closely collaborate; under such circumstances, many of these persons
are successfully treated.

The Role of the Police. A large proportion of acutely mentally ill persons
come first to the attention of the police (McNiel and others, 1991; Zealberg
and others, 1992; Way, Evans, and Banks, 1993; Lamb and others, 1995).
Even if the police consider the problem to be mental illness, the mental
health option can involve a number of problems and irritants. There may
be long waiting periods in emergency rooms during which police officers
cannot attend to other duties. Mental health professionals may question the
judgment of police and refuse admission, or they may admit for only a brief
hospital stay a person who just a short time before constituted a clear men-

ace to the community (Laberge and Morin, 1995; Lamb and others, 1984; Rogers, 1990).

On the other hand, the police know very well that if they refer a psychiatric case to the criminal justice system, the offender will be dealt with in a more systematic way. He or she will be taken into custody, will probably be seen by a mental health professional attached to the court or in the jail, and will probably receive psychiatric evaluation and treatment. Thus, arrest is a response with which police are familiar, one over which they have more control, and one that they believe will lead to an appropriate disposition (Laberge and Morin, 1995; Holley and Arboleda-Florez, 1988). Moreover, when persons who are socially disruptive are excluded from psychiatric facilities, the criminal justice system becomes the system "that can't say no" (Borzecki and Wormith, 1985, p. 243).

With regard to minor offenses, a number of factors have been proposed to explain why a mentally ill person is arrested rather than taken to a hospital. A person who appears mentally ill to a mental health professional may not appear so to police officers, who, despite their practical experience, have not had sufficient training in dealing with this population and are still laypersons in these matters (Husted and Nehemkis, 1995; Husted, Charter, and Perrou, 1995). Also, mental illness may appear to the police as simply alcohol or drug intoxication, especially if the mentally ill person has been using drugs or alcohol at the time of arrest. Still another factor is that in the heat and confusion of an encounter with the police and other citizens, which may include forcibly subduing the offender, signs of mental illness may go unnoticed (Lamb and Grant, 1982).

In addition, law enforcement officers may be more inclined to take mentally ill persons to jail if they believe no appropriate community alternatives are available (Ogloff and Otto, 1989), a practice that has been referred to as *mercy booking*. Although this practice may be viewed as unconstitutional, the vast majority of states have not enacted legislation against detaining noncriminal mentally ill people in jail (Ogloff and others, 1990).

The demands of citizens also come into play. Many retail stores have a policy that anyone caught shoplifting should go to jail, and store managers are instructed to make a citizen's arrest and call the police without exception. In another kind of situation, people who have just been assaulted by a psychotic person are frequently not inclined to be sympathetic to their assailant even when mental disturbance is evident. Thus, an angry citizen may insist on signing a citizen's arrest and having the person taken to jail.

Society's Attitudes. The public has traditionally believed that any sentence other than prison is too lenient for serious offenders, even if they are mentally ill (Petersilia, 1987). Moreover, some view mental illness as volitional and perhaps a deliberate attempt to avoid punishment (Perr, 1985; Johnson, 1985). Still another important factor is the public's fear of mentally ill persons who commit criminal offenses.

The public's growing intolerance of perpetrators, whether mentally ill or not, is demonstrated by its acceptance of and desire for more restrictive detention laws for offenders. With respect to offenders with mental disorders, some states have repealed sexual psychopathology laws that permitted mental health treatment for sex offenders rather than criminal processing and imprisonment. Diminished capacity, which can be a factor in granting a more lenient sentence, has also been repealed in a number of states. Moreover, legislation has been passed whereby offenders with mental disorders in prison can have their periods of social control extended if they are identified as dangerous before their parole date or the expiration of their sentence. For example, in California, mentally ill offenders considered to be dangerous (California Penal Code, sec. 2962) and sexually violent predators (California Welfare and Institutions Code, sec. 6600) are usually transferred on their parole date or on expiration of their sentence to state mental hospitals, where they are confined for treatment for renewable periods of one or two years. In our opinion, these laws reflect the attitudes of society toward mentally ill offenders.

Although psychiatric interventions exist in the criminal justice system, mentally ill persons are more strictly controlled in that system than are patients in psychiatric hospitals (Laberge and Morin, 1995). Moreover, the criminal justice system, despite protestations to the contrary, appears to have little interest in decriminalizing persons with psychiatric disorders even though they represent a considerable burden and use scarce resources. In a thoughtful article, Laberge and Morin (1995) observed that a general decriminalization of psychiatric cases would threaten the criminal justice system to its foundations because such an approach might be perceived as undermining the principle of equality of all before the law. This perception would exist even where criminal law recognizes mental disorders as conferring a special status.

Specific treatment of mentally ill persons in the criminal justice system is often seen as special treatment both by the general public and within the criminal justice system. For instance, the insanity defense is perceived by most Americans as a frequently raised defense, as well as a way to evade justice. However, studies have shown that this defense is seldom used and rarely successful (Pasewark and Pantle, 1981; Sales and Hafemeister, 1984). In addition, it has been demonstrated that persons who successfully use this defense may be detained for considerably longer periods than others convicted for the same offenses (Pasewark, 1986; Golding, Eaves, and Kowaz, 1989).

Moreover, it appears the criminal justice system is more inclined to interpret and deal with criminal behavior in terms of illness when the deviant person acknowledges the illness and is willing to undergo treatment for it (Conrad and Schneider, 1980). Clearly, the appropriateness of treating mentally ill offenders safely in the community should be assessed. However, undertaking successful treatment for this population can be daunting.

For instance, Brelje (1985) wrote that effective psychotherapy for mentally ill offenders involves the patient's insight, an awareness of vulnerability to or presence of a mental disorder, a realistic understanding of the nature of the mental illness, a motivation to change or prevent recurrence of symptoms, an acceptance of treatment goals and strategies, realistic personal goals, and the patient's awareness of his or her legal status and its meaning.

However, Laberge and Morin (1957) have observed that many mentally ill offenders do not take responsibility for their illness or their offenses and do not acknowledge their need for treatment. They refuse a therapeutic relationship and refuse to take medication and keep appointments. Therefore, they are often not seen by society as persons who should be excused for their legal transgressions. It appears that despite the concern of mental health professionals and many family members about mentally ill persons in jail, the general public would show little support for not placing social controls on individuals who commit offenses and refuse to submit to treatment that sets limits on their behavior.

Thus, criminalization of mentally ill persons who have committed minor offenses cannot be seen as resulting simply from the usual explanations of lack of long-term hospitalization, lack of adequate support systems in the community, difficulty in gaining entry into the mental health system, and more restrictive criteria for civil commitment. Another crucial factor is society's concern that criminal offenses be dealt with and that persons committing them be controlled and punished, especially if they are not clearly willing to accept the patient role.

Conclusion and Recommendations

Much has been learned about what needs to be done to prevent mentally ill persons from being inappropriately placed in the criminal justice system and about how to treat them once they are there and after they are released into the community. What has been lacking is widespread and comprehensive implementation of interventions shown to be effective (Jamelka, Rahman, and Trupin, 1993). Several of these strategies are summarized below.

Steps should be taken to prevent inappropriate arrest of mentally ill persons (Husted, 1994). The police are often the first to respond to emergencies involving people with severe psychiatric disturbances (Zealberg and others, 1992). However, the police may not always recognize a need for, or have access to, emergency psychiatric resources. Clearly, mental health expertise is needed at this point to prevent criminalization. There is a pressing need for formal training of police officers to help them better understand mental illness and improve their attitudes toward individuals with mental disorders (Husted, Charter, and Perrou, 1995; Murphy, 1989).

Mental health consultation provided to the police in the field can result in a response that combines the specialized knowledge and expertise of law enforcement and mental health professionals. Such an approach can greatly increase the number of mentally ill persons given appropriate access to the mental health system rather than inappropriately diverted to the criminal justice system. For example, an evaluation of psychiatric emergency teams consisting of police officers and mental health professionals found that the teams were able to deal with psychiatric emergencies in the field, even with a population characterized by acute and chronic severe mental illness, a high potential for violence, a high prevalence of serious substance abuse, and long histories with both the criminal justice and the mental health systems (Lamb and others, 1995). These teams took or sent almost all of the persons in crisis to the mental health system and not to jail.

For individuals who are arrested and placed in jail, it is generally recommended that the facility routinely screen all incoming detainees for severe mental disorder and that jail administrators negotiate programmatic relationships with mental health agencies to provide multidisciplinary psychiatric teams (Teplin, 1990; Lamb and others, 1984). These teams should be established inside jails to provide short-term crisis evaluation, treatment, and referral to a psychiatric hospital if necessary. The teams should include psychiatrists so that psychoactive medications can be prescribed.

Mentally ill detainees who have committed minor crimes, such as trespassing and disorderly conduct, should be diverted to the mental health system entirely, or at minimum for treatment. For instance, mental health teams should be readily available for consultation to the arraignment courts and especially to the municipal courts, where many acutely psychotic patients appear with very minimal criminal charges. Steadman, Barbera, and Dennis (1994) found that only a small number of U.S. jails have diversion programs for mentally ill detainees. They also observed that objective data on the effectiveness of these programs are lacking. On the other hand, it has been found that court-mandated and -monitored treatment in lieu of jail was effective in obtaining a good outcome for chronically and severely mentally ill persons who committed misdemeanors (Lamb, Weinberger, and Reston-Parham, 1996).

Belcher (1988) wrote that a system that relies solely on voluntary compliance may not provide adequate structure for mentally ill offenders. He and others (Torrey, 1997; Husted, 1994; Swanson and others, 1997a; Hoffman, 1990; Miller, 1992; Clear, Byrne, and Dvoskin, 1993) recommended such mechanisms as outpatient commitment, court-monitored treatment, treatment as a condition of probation or parole, and psychiatric conservatorship or supervision by agencies such as Oregon's Psychiatric Security Review Board (Rogers, Bloom, and Manson, 1982). Freeman and Roesch (1989) acknowledged that the court or parole board has a right to set conditions for release to the community that include mandatory treatment. Nevertheless, mental health professionals have an ethical and legal obligation to inform patients fully about the nature of the treatment and obtain their consent for it.

It is important to recognize that persons with mental disorders who are discharged from psychiatric or correctional institutions experience multiple problems that cannot be adequately treated in traditional community-based facilities (Stein and Test, 1980; Witheridge and Dincin, 1985). Thus, placement in the community often results in rehospitalization or reincarceration (Lamb and Weinberger, 1993). To reduce this cycle, assertive case management programs are recommended.

The great majority of mentally ill offenders need the basic elements of case management, which starts with the premise that each person has a designated professional with overall responsibility for his or her care (Dvoskin and Steadman, 1994; Lamb and Weinberger, 1993). The case manager formulates an individualized treatment and rehabilitation plan with the participation of the mentally ill person and often the supervision of the court. As care progresses, the case manager monitors the mentally ill person to determine if he or she is receiving and complying with treatment, has an appropriate living situation, has adequate funds, and has access to vocational rehabilitation.

The case manager not only provides outreach services, but also serves as an advocate for the individual and makes sure that the mentally ill person is not drifting away from the supportive elements of such a network. An assertive case management program deals with clients on a frequent and long-term basis, using a hands-on approach that may necessitate meeting with clients on their own turf or even seeing clients daily (Wilson, Tien, and Eaves, 1995). This form of contact and familiarity with clients helps the case manager and client anticipate and prevent significant decompensation.

Important advances have been made in recent years in the management of the violent behavior of severely mentally ill persons (Harris and Rice, 1997; Buckley and others, 1997). Behavior therapy and pharmacotherapy—in particular, the use of the new atypical antipsychotic medications—are but a few examples. It is crucial that these modalities be widely implemented.

Mental health agencies in the community must be able to provide the degree of structure and limit setting needed by mentally ill offenders, as well as ensure the safety of staff. When highly structured twenty-four-hour care is required, it should be provided.

The role of family members is an important aspect in the care of mentally ill offenders. Often overlooked are family members' needs for guidance and support. Families should be instructed in ways to help stabilize their relative (Lamb and Weinberger, 1993). They should also be involved in support programs to help them during crises and in self-help programs so they can benefit from the experience of other families in similar situations (Hylton, 1995).

We believe that a significant increase in mental health services for severely mentally ill persons, from outpatient treatment and case management to highly structured twenty-four-hour care, would result in far fewer mentally ill persons' committing criminal offenses. Thus, one of our most important recommendations is for increased mental health services. The criminal justice system should not be viewed as an appropriate substitute for the mental health system. Moreover, it has been our experience that an enormous stigma is attached to people who have been categorized as both mentally ill and an offender, and it is thus extremely difficult to place them in community treatment and housing. The difficulty is even greater when they have been in a forensic hospital.

Clearly, many mentally ill persons who commit criminal offenses present formidable challenges to treatment because of their treatment resistance, poor compliance with antipsychotic medications, potential dangerousness, high rate of substance abuse, and need for structure. To a large extent, the public mental health system has given up on them and allowed them to become the responsibility of the criminal justice system. We believe these recommendations would contribute to successful treatment of this population.

Implementing these recommendations would mean tailoring mental health services to meet the needs of mentally ill offenders and not treating them as if they were compliant, cooperative, and in need of a minimum of controls. The lives of a large proportion are characterized by chaos, dysphoria, and deprivation as they try to survive in a world for which they are ill prepared. They cry out for treatment and for structure, and we believe it is the obligation of the mental health system to provide it. If effective and appropriate interventions are provided, these individuals may not only improve psychiatrically but may also engage in considerably less criminal behavior.

References

Abramson, M. F. "The Criminalization of Mentally Disordered Behavior: Possible Side-Effects of a New Mental Health Law." *Hospital and Community Psychiatry*, 1972, *23*, 101–105.

Alaska. Alaska Statutes 47.30.740.

American Bar Association, Criminal Justice Standards Committee. *ABA Criminal Justice Mental Health Standards*. Washington, D.C.: American Bar Association, Criminal Justice Standards Committee, 1986.

Appelbaum, P. S. "Almost a Revolution: An International Perspective on the Law of Involuntary Commitment." *Journal of the American Academy of Psychiatry and the Law*, 1997, *25*, 135–147.

Arthur Bolton Associates. *Report to the California State Legislature*. Sacramento, Calif.: Arthur Bolton Associates, Oct. 1976.

Arvanites, K. "The Impact of State Mental Hospital Deinstitutionalization on Commitments for Incompetency to Stand Trial." *Criminology*, 1988, *26*, 307–320.

Bachrach, L. L., Talbott, J. A., and Meyerson, A. T. "The Chronic Psychiatric Patient as a 'Difficult' Patient: A Conceptual Analysis." In A. T. Meyerson (ed.), *Barriers to Treating the Chronic Mentally Ill*. New Directions for Mental Health Services, no 33. San Francisco: Jossey-Bass, 1987.

Belcher, J. R. "Are Jails Replacing the Mental Health System for the Homeless Mentally Ill?" *Community Mental Health Journal*, 1988, *24*, 185–195.

Borzecki, M., and Wormith, J. S. "The Criminalization of Psychiatrically Ill People: A Review with a Canadian Perspective." *Psychiatric Journal of the University of Ottawa*, 1985, *1*, 241–247.

Brelje, T. B. "Problems of Treatment of NGRIs in an Inpatient Mental Health System." Paper presented at a meeting of the Illinois Association of Community Mental Health Agencies, Chicago, 1985.

Buckley, P. F., and others. "Aggression and Schizophrenia: Efficacy of Risperidone." *Journal of the American Academy of Psychiatry and the Law*, 1997, *25*, 173–181.

California. California Penal Code, sec. 2962.

California. California Welfare and Institutions Code, sec. 5300.

California, California Welfare and Institutions Code, sec. 6600.

Clear, T. R., Byrne, J. M., and Dvoskin, J. A. "The Transition from Being an Inmate: Discharge Planning, Parole, and Community-Based Services for Offenders with Mental Illness." In H. J. Steadman and J. J. Cocozza (eds.), *Mental Illness in America's Prisons*. Seattle, Wash.: National Coalition for the Mentally Ill in the Criminal Justice System, 1993.

Cocozza, J. J., Steadman, H. J., and Melick, M. E. "Trends in Violent Crime Among Ex–Mental Patients." *Criminology*, 1978, *16*, 317–334.

Conrad, P., and Schneider, J. W. *Deviance and Medicalization: From Badness to Sickness.* St. Louis, Mo.: Mosby–Year Book, 1980.

Davis, S. "Assessing the 'Criminalization' of the Mentally Ill in Canada." *Canadian Journal of Psychiatry*, 1992, *37*, 532–538.

Dickey, W. "Incompetency and the Nondangerous Mentally Ill Client." *Criminal Law Bulletin*, 1980, *16*, 22–40.

Draine, J., Solomon, P., and Meyerson, A. T. "Predictors of Reincarceration Among Patients Who Received Psychiatric Services in Jail." *Hospital and Community Psychiatry*, 1994, *45*, 163–167.

Dvoskin, J. A., and Steadman, H. J. "Using Intensive Case Management to Reduce Violence by Mentally Ill Persons in the Community." *Hospital and Community Psychiatry*, 1994, *45*, 679–684.

Freeman, R. J., and Roesch, R. "Mental Disorder and the Criminal Justice System: A Review." *International Journal of Law and Psychiatry*, 1989, *12*, 105–115.

Fulwiler, C., and others. "Early-Onset Substance Abuse and Community Violence by Outpatients with Chronic Mental Illness." *Psychiatric Services*, 1997, *48*, 1181–1185.

Gibbs, J. J. "Problems and Priorities: Perceptions of Jail Custodians and Social Service Providers." *Journal of Criminal Justice*, 1983, *11*, 327–349.

Golding, S., Eaves, D., and Kowaz, A. "The Assessment, Treatment, and Community Outcome of Insanity Acquitees: Forensic History and Response to Treatment." *International Journal of Law and Psychiatry*, 1989, *12*, 149–179.

Grunberg, F., Klinger, B. I., and Grument, B. R. "Homicide and the Deinstitutionalization of the Mentally Ill." *American Journal of Psychiatry*, 1977, *134*, 685–687.

Guy, E., and others. "Mental Health Status of Prisoners in an Urban Jail." *Criminal Justice and Behavior*, 1985, *12*, 29–53.

Harris, G. T., and Rice, M. E. "Risk Appraisal and Management of Violent Behavior." *Psychiatric Services*, 1997,*48*, 1168–1176.

Hochstedler, E. "Criminal Prosecution of the Mentally Disordered." *Law and Society Review*, 1986, *20*, 279–292.

Hochstedler, E. "Twice-Cursed? The Mentally Disordered Defendant." *Criminal Justice and Behavior*, 1987, *14*, 251–267.

Hodgins, S. "Mental Disorder, Intellectual Deficiency, and Crime: Evidence from a Birth Cohort." *Archives of General Psychiatry*, 1992, *49*, 476–483.

Hodgins, S., and others. "Mental Disorder and Crime: Evidence from a Danish Birth Cohort." *Archives of General Psychiatry*, 1996, *53*, 489–496.

Hoffman, B. F. "The Criminalization of the Mentally Ill." *Canadian Journal of Psychiatry*, 1990, *35*, 166–169.

Holley, H. L., and Arboleda-Florez, J. "Criminalization of the Mentally Ill: I. Police Perceptions." *Canadian Journal of Psychiatry*, 1988, *33*, 81–86.

Husted, J. R. "The Last Asylum: The Mentally Ill Offender in the Criminal Justice System." In D. T. Marsh (ed.), *New Directions in the Psychological Treatment of Serious Mental Illness.* New York: Praeger, 1994.

Husted, J. R., Charter, R. A., and Perrou, M. A. "California Law Enforcement Agencies and the Mentally Ill Offender." *Bulletin of the American Academy of Psychiatry and the Law,* 1995, *23,* 315–329.

Husted, J., and Nehemkis, A. "Civil Commitment Viewed from Three Perspectives: Professional, Family, and Police." *Bulletin of the American Academy of Psychiatry and the Law,* 1995, *23,* 533–546.

Hylton, J. H. "Care or Control: Health or Criminal Justice Options for the Long-Term Seriously Mentally Ill in a Canadian Province." *International Journal of Law and Psychiatry,* 1995, *18,* 45–59.

Jemelka, R. P., Rahman, S., and Trupin, E. W. "Prison Mental Health: An Overview." In H. J. Steadman and J. J. Cocozza (eds.), *Mental Illness in America's Prisons.* Seattle, Wash.: National Coalition for the Mentally Ill in the Criminal Justice System, 1993.

Jemelka, R. P., Trupin, E. W., and Chiles, J. A. "The Mentally Ill in Prisons: A Review." *Hospital and Community Psychiatry,* 1989, *40,* 481–491.

Jemelka, R. P., and others. "Computerized Offender Assessment: Validation Study." *Psychological Assessment,* 1992, *4,* 138–144.

Johnson, P. E. "The Turnabout in the Insanity Defense." In M. Tonry and N. Morris (eds.), *Crime and Justice: An Annual Review of Research.* Chicago: University of Chicago Press, 1985.

Junginger, J. "Psychosis and Violence: The Case for a Content Analysis of Psychotic Experience." *Schizophrenia Bulletin,* 1996, *22,* 91–103.

Kanter, J. (ed.). *Clinical Studies in Case Management.* New Directions for Mental Health Services, no. 65. San Francisco: Jossey-Bass, 1995.

Laberge, D., and Morin, D. "The Overuse of Criminal Justice Dispositions: Failure of Diversionary Policies in the Management of Mental Health Problems." *International Journal of Law and Psychiatry,* 1995, *18,* 389–414.

Lamb, H. R. *Treating the Long-Term Mentally Ill.* San Francisco: Jossey-Bass, 1982.

Lamb, H. R. "Incompetency to Stand Trial: Appropriateness and Outcome." *Archives of General Psychiatry,* 1987, *44,* 754–758.

Lamb, H. R. "The New State Mental Hospitals in the Community." *Psychiatric Services,* 1997, *48,* 1307–1310.

Lamb, H. R. "Public Psychiatry and Prevention." In R. E. Hales, S. C. Yudofsky, and J. A. (eds.), *Textbook of Psychiatry.* (3rd ed.) Washington, D.C.: American Psychiatric Press, 1999.

Lamb, H. R., and Grant, R. W. "The Mentally Ill in an Urban County Jail." *Archives of General Psychiatry,* 1982, *39,* 17–22.

Lamb, H. R., and Grant, R. W. "Mentally Ill Women in a County Jail." *Archives of General Psychiatry,* 1983, *40,* 363–368.

Lamb, H. R., and Mills, M. J. "Needed Changes in Law and Procedure for the Chronically Mentally Ill." *Hospital and Community Psychiatry,* 1986, *37,* 475–480.

Lamb, H. R., and Weinberger, L. E. "Therapeutic Use of Conservatorship in the Treatment of Gravely Disabled Psychiatric Patients." *Hospital and Community Psychiatry,* 1993, *44,* 147–150.

Lamb, H. R., Weinberger, L. E., and Reston-Parham, C. "Court Intervention to Address the Mental Health Needs of Mentally Ill Offenders." *Psychiatric Services,* 1996, *47,* 275–281.

Lamb, H. R., and others. "Psychiatric Needs in Local Jails: Emergency Issues." *American Journal of Psychiatry,* 1984, *141,* 774–777.

Lamb, H. R., and others. "Outcome for Psychiatric Emergency Patients Seen by an Outreach Police–Mental Health Team." *Psychiatric Services,* 1995, *4,* 1267–1271.

Link, B. G., and Stueve, A. "Evidence Bearing on Mental Illness as a Possible Cause of Violent Behavior." *Epidemiological Review,* 1995, *17,* 172–181.

Martell, D. A., Rosner, R., and Harmon, R. B. "Base-Rate Estimates of Criminal Behavior by Homeless Mentally Ill Persons in New York City." *Psychiatric Services,* 1995, *46,* 596–600.

Marzuk, P. M. "Violence, Crime, and Mental Illness: How Strong a Link?" *Archives of General Psychiatry,* 1996, *53,* 481–486.

McNiel, D. E., and others. "Characteristics of Persons Referred by Police to the Psychiatric Emergency Room." *Hospital and Community Psychiatry,* 1991, *42,* 425–427.

Mednick, S. A., Brennan, P., and Katila, H. "Mental Illness, Violence, and Fetal Neural Development." Paper presented at the annual meeting of the American Psychiatric Association, New York, May 4–9, 1996.

Michaels, D., and others. "Homelessness and Indicators of Mental Illness Among Inmates in New York City's Correctional System." *Hospital and Community Psychiatry,* 1992, *43,* 150–155.

Miller, R. D. "An Update on Involuntary Civil Commitment to Outpatient Treatment." *Hospital and Community Psychiatry,* 1992, *43,* 79–81.

Monahan, J. "Mental Disorder and Violent Behavior." *American Psychologist,* 1992, *47,* 511–521.

Mulvey, E. P. "Assessing the Evidence of a Link Between Mental Illness and Violence." *Hospital and Community Psychiatry,* 1994, *45,* 663–668.

Murphy, G. R. *Managing Persons with Mental Disabilities: A Curriculum Guide for Police Trainers.* Washington, D.C.: Police Executive Research Forum, 1989.

Neighbors, H. W. "The Prevalence of Mental Disorder in Michigan Prisons." *DIS Newsletter* [Department of Psychiatry, Washington University School of Medicine, St. Louis], 1987, *7,* 8–11.

Ogloff, R. P., and Otto, R. K. "Mental Health Interventions in Jails." In P. Keller and S. Heyman (eds.), *Innovations in Clinical Practice.* Sarasota, Fla.: Professional Resource Exchange, 1989.

Ogloff, R. P., and others. "Preventing the Detention of Non-Criminal Mentally Ill People in Jails: The Need for Emergency Protective Custody Units." *Nebraska Law Review,* 1990, *69,* 434–471.

Palermo, G. B., Smith, M. B., and Liska, F. J. "Jails Versus Mental Hospitals: A Social Dilemma." *International Journal of Offender Therapy and Comparative Criminology,* 1991, *35,* 97–106.

Pasewark, R. A. "A Review of Research on the Insanity Defense." *Annals of the American Academy of Political and Social Science,* 1986, *484,* 100–114.

Pasewark, R. A., and Pantle, M. "Opinions About the Insanity Plea." *Journal of Forensic Psychology,* 1981, *8,* 63–67.

Penrose, L. "Mental Disease and Crime: Outline of a Comparative Study of European Statistics." *British Journal of Medical Psychology,* 1939, *18,* 1–15.

Perr, I. N. "The Insanity Defense: The Case for Abolition." *Hospital and Community Psychiatry,* 1985, *36,* 51–54.

Petersilia, J. *Expanding Options for Criminal Sentencing.* Santa Monica, Calif.: Rand, 1987.

Rogers, A. "Policing Mental Disorder: Controversies, Myths, and Realities." *Social Policy and Administration,* 1990, *24,* 226–236.

Rogers, J. L., Bloom, J. D., and Manson, S. "Oregon's Innovative System for Supervising Offenders Found Not Guilty by Reason of Insanity." *Hospital and Community Psychiatry,* 1982, *33,* 1022–1023.

Sales, B., and Hafemeister, T. "Empiricism and Legal Policy on the Insanity Defense." In L. Teplin (ed.), *Mental Health and Criminal Justice.* Thousand Oaks, Calif.: Sage, 1984.

Schuerman, L. A., and Kobrin, S. "Exposure of Community Mental Health Clients to the Criminal Justice System: Client/Criminal or Patient/Prisoner." In L. Teplin (ed.), *Mental Health and Criminal Justice.* Thousand Oaks, Calif.: Sage, 1984.

Sosowsky, L. "Crime and Violence Among Mental Patients Reconsidered in View of the New Legal Relationship Between the State and the Mentally Ill." *American Journal of Psychiatry,* 1978, *135,* 33–42.

Sosowsky, L. "Explaining the Increased Arrest Rate Among Mental Patients: A Cautionary Note." *American Journal of Psychiatry*, 1980, *137*, 1602–1605.

Steadman, H. J. "Risk Factors for Community Violence Among Acute Psychiatric Inpatients: The MacArthur Risk Assessment Project." Paper presented at the annual meeting of the American Psychiatric Association, San Diego, May 17–22, 1997.

Steadman, H. J., Barbera, S. S., and Dennis, D. L. "A National Survey of Jail Diversion Programs for Mentally Ill Detainees." *Hospital and Community Psychiatry*, 1994, *45*, 1109–1113.

Steadman, H. J., Cocozza, J. J., and Melick, M. E. "Explaining the Increased Arrest Rate Among Mental Patients: The Changing Clientele of State Hospitals." *American Journal of Psychiatry*, 1978, *135*, 816–820.

Steadman, H. J., Vanderwyst, D., and Ribner, S. "Comparing Arrest Rates of Mental Patients and Criminal Offenders." *American Journal of Psychiatry*, 1978, *135*, 1218–1224.

Steadman, H. J., and others. "The Impact of State Mental Hospital Deinstitutionalization on United States Prison Populations, 1968–1978." *Journal of Criminal Law and Criminology*, 1984, *75*, 474–490.

Steadman, H. J., and others. "A Survey of Mental Disability Among State Prison Inmates." *Hospital and Community Psychiatry*, 1987, *38*, 1086–1090.

Stein, L. I., and Test, M. A. "Alternative to Mental Hospital Treatment." *Archives of General Psychiatry*, 1980, *37*, 392–397.

Stelovich, S. "From the Hospital to the Prison: A Step Forward in Deinstitutionalization?" *Hospital and Community Psychiatry*, 1979, *30*, 618–620.

Steury, E. H. "Specifying 'Criminalization' of the Mentally Disordered Misdemeanant." *Journal of Criminal Law and Criminology*, 1991, *82*, 334–359.

Stone, A. A. "Comment." *American Journal of Psychiatry*, 1978, *135*, 61–63.

Stone, M. H. "Criminality and Psychopathology." *Journal of Practical Psychiatry and Behavioral Health*, 1997, *3*, 146–155.

Survey and Analysis Branch, Center for Mental Health Services. *Resident Patients in State and County Mental Hospitals, 1998 Survey.* Washington, D.C.: Substance Abuse and Mental Health Services Administration, U.S. Department of Health and Human Services, 2000.

Swank, G., and Winer, D. "Occurrence of Psychiatric Disorders in a County Jail Population." *American Journal of Psychiatry*, 1976, *133*, 1331–1333.

Swanson, J. W., and others. "Interpreting the Effectiveness of Involuntary Outpatient Commitment: A Conceptual Model." *Journal of the American Academy of Psychiatry and the Law*, 1997a, *25*, 5–16.

Swanson, J. W., and others. "Violence and Severe Mental Disorder in Clinical and Community Populations: The Effects of Psychotic Symptoms, Comorbidity, and Lack of Treatment." *Psychiatry*, 1997b, *60*, 1–22.

Teplin, L. A. "The Criminalization of the Mentally Ill: Speculation in Search of Data." *Psychological Bulletin*, 1983, *94*, 54–67.

Teplin, L. A. "Criminalizing Mental Disorder: The Comparative Arrest Rate of the Mentally Ill." *American Psychologist*, 1984, *39*, 794–803.

Teplin, L. A. "The Prevalence of Severe Mental Disorder Among Male Urban Jail Detainees: Comparison with the Epidemiologic Catchment Area Program." *American Journal of Public Health*, 1990, *80*, 663–669.

Teplin, L. A., Abram, K. M., and McClelland, G. M. "Prevalence of Psychiatric Disorders Among Incarcerated Women." *Archives of General Psychiatry*, 1996, *53*, 505–512.

Torrey, E. F. "Violent Behavior by Individuals with Serious Mental Illness." *Hospital and Community Psychiatry*, 1994, *4*, 653–662.

Torrey, E. F. *Out of the Shadows: Confronting America's Mental Illness Crisis.* New York: Wiley, 1997.

U.S. Department of Justice, Bureau of Justice Statistics. *State and Federal Prisons Report Record Growth During Last Twelve Months.* Washington, D.C.: U.S. Department of Justice, Bureau of Justice Statistics, Dec. 1995.

Washington. Revised Code of Washington Annotated (West), sec. 71.05.280.

Way, B. B., Evans, M. E., and Banks, S. M. "An Analysis of Police Referrals to 10 Psychiatric Emergency Rooms." *Bulletin of the American Academy of Psychiatry and the Law*, 1993, *21*, 389–396.

Whitmer, G. E. "From Hospitals to Jails: The Fate of California's Deinstitutionalized Mentally Ill." *American Journal of Orthopsychiatry*, 1980, *50*, 65–75.

Wilson, D., Tien, G., and Eaves, D. "Increasing the Community Tenure of Mentally Disordered Offenders: An Assertive Case Management Program." *International Journal of Law and Psychiatry*, 1995, *18*, 61–69.

Witheridge, T. F., and Dincin, J. "The Bridge: An Assertive Outreach Program in an Urban Setting." In L. I. Stein and M. A. Test (eds.), *The Training in Community Living Model: A Decade of Experience.* New Directions for Mental Health Services, no 26. San Francisco: Jossey-Bass, 1985.

Zealberg, J. J., and others. "A Mobile Crisis Program: Collaboration Between Emergency Psychiatric Services and Police." *Hospital and Community Psychiatry*, 1992, *43*, 612–615.

Zitrin, A., and others. "Crime and Violence Among Mental Patients." *American Journal of Psychiatry*, 1976, *133*, 142–149.

H. RICHARD LAMB is professor of psychiatry and the behavioral sciences at Keck School of Medicine, University of Southern California, in Los Angeles.

LINDA E. WEINBERGER is professor of clinical psychiatry and chief psychologist at the Institute of Psychiatry, Law, and Behavioral Sciences at Keck School of Medicine, University of Southern California, in Los Angeles.

4

Community treatment of severely mentally ill offenders who fall under the jurisdiction of the criminal justice system has important differences from treatment of non-offenders. It is critical to identify a treatment philosophy that strikes a balance between individual rights and public safety and includes clear treatment goals.

Community Treatment of Severely Mentally Ill Offenders Under the Jurisdiction of the Criminal Justice System: A Review

H. Richard Lamb, Linda E. Weinberger, Bruce H. Gross

The treatment of severely mentally ill offenders in the community has become an increasingly important and urgent issue because of the greatly increased numbers of persons with severe mental illness who have found their way into the criminal justice system. Factors cited as causes for these increases are deinstitutionalization, more rigid criteria for civil commitment, lack of adequate community support for persons with mental illness, mentally ill offenders' difficulty gaining access to community mental health treatment, violence at the time of arrest, and the attitudes of police officers and society (Borzecki and Wormith, 1985; Jemelka, Trupin, and Chiles, 1989; Robertson, Pearson, and Gibb, 1996; Lamb and Weinberger, 1998).

This chapter reviews the literature on community treatment of severely mentally ill offenders and discusses the principles of treating this population as generally viewed by clinicians in forensic mental health care who conduct such treatment and by the criminal justice system under whose jurisdiction the treatment occurs. Many mental health professionals who previously may not have been involved in treating mentally ill offenders are now finding themselves with treatment responsibilities for this population. A need exists for a clear understanding of the criminal justice system's perspectives and goals related to the treatment of mentally ill offenders. The perspectives and goals include an emphasis on concerns about public safety, control of violence, extensive use of authority, and close cooperation between the mental health and criminal justice systems (Hafemeister and Petrila, 1994; Morris, 1997).

Source: Lamb, H. R., Weinberger, L. E., and Gross, B. H. "Community Treatment of Severely Mentally Ill Offenders Under the Jurisdiction of the Criminal Justice System: A Review." *Psychiatric Services,* 1999, *50* (7), 907–913. Reprinted by permission.

Community treatment of mentally ill offenders is conducted under a variety of circumstances. This chapter focuses on offenders who remain under the jurisdiction of the criminal justice system. One such group consists of individuals given probation by the court that includes a condition of mandatory outpatient treatment. Another consists of individuals referred for treatment by their parole officer with the understanding that failure to comply may result in a revocation of parole and return to custody. In addition, some offenders are diverted by the court from the criminal justice system to the mental health system; the prosecution of their case may be postponed by the judge until they successfully complete a specified treatment program, at which time criminal charges are dismissed.

Although practices vary from state to state, offenders who are acquitted as not guilty by reason of insanity are often placed in mandatory outpatient treatment (conditional release programs), as are persons found incompetent to stand trial and persons who fall under the jurisdiction of laws regarding dangerous mentally ill offenders. Another category of offenders who may be given outpatient treatment are sex offenders. Although a number of states have sexual psychopathology laws related to the treatment of these persons, a discussion of such treatment is beyond the scope of this chapter.

Methods

MEDLINE, *Psychological Abstracts,* and the *Index to Legal Periodicals and Books* were searched from 1978, and all pertinent references were obtained.

Results

Treatment Within a Criminal Justice Context. Both the mentally ill offender and the therapist must satisfy legal requirements, such as regular attendance and periodic progress reports. The patient must comply with legal restrictions, such as abstinence from drugs and alcohol. Moreover, mentally ill offenders must come to terms with the fact that they have committed an illegal act and that they have been judged to have a psychiatric disorder and to need treatment.

Both the criminal justice system and forensic clinicians generally expect that mentally ill offenders given treatment will gain some understanding of the role of their psychiatric disorder in past and potential future dangerous behavior and that they will avoid behavior or situations that might increase the risk for criminal activity or a deterioration in their clinical condition (Wasyliw, Cavanaugh, and Grossman, 1988; Miraglia and Giglio, 1993; Dvoskin and Steadman, 1994). Moreover, both society and the criminal justice system expect that treatment will be conducted under conditions that can, to the greatest extent possible, ensure public safety.

Thus, a balance must exist among individual rights, the need for treatment, and public safety (Wasyliw, Cavanaugh, and Grossman, 1988; Griffin, Steadman, and Heilbrun, 1991; Heilbrun and Griffin, 1998). However, it has been argued that courts place a greater emphasis on the potential dangerousness of the mentally ill offender than on the individual's rights (Hafemeister and Petrila, 1994; Morris, 1997). In so doing, the courts place the burden on the mentally ill offender to demonstrate that he or she no longer poses a danger to the community.

Outpatient treatment for severely mentally ill offenders is not designed to make currently dangerous individuals nondangerous. Rather, the criminal justice system presumes that mentally ill offenders placed in outpatient treatment will not be dangerous to others while under supervision and treatment in the community. A primary concern in outpatient treatment of these individuals is to assess any changes in mental condition that may indicate dangerousness and to reduce potential threat of harm. Therefore, features that contribute to a patient's risk of harm are addressed first in treatment. Miraglia and Giglio (1993) note that "an ability to assess dangerousness and to incorporate this assessment into an intervention strategy is the single most important skill for the outpatient clinician to possess" (p. 233). Thus, clinicians must have as great as possible an understanding of each patient's potential for violence as a function of his or her history and psychiatric condition (Bullard, 1994; Cohen and Eastman, 1997).

In contrast, in nonforensic psychiatric treatment, the primary focus is usually on alleviation of symptoms. Clinicians who treat mentally ill offenders need to recognize that they have assumed responsibility not only to the patient but to society in ensuring the patient's safety to the community. This responsibility is not as central when clinicians are treating nonoffenders.

Challenges of Community Treatment of Mentally Ill Offenders. Severely mentally ill individuals who have committed criminal offenses represent a challenge to outpatient clinicians. The problem lies not only in ensuring safety to the community but in working with individuals who may be resistant to treatment (Heilbrun and Griffin, 1998).

A large proportion of severely mentally ill persons who commit criminal offenses have a history of being highly resistant to psychiatric treatment before their involvement in the criminal justice system (Lamb, 1987; Laberge and Morin, 1995). They may have refused referral, may not have kept appointments, may not have been compliant with psychoactive medications, and may have refused appropriate housing placements. Problems of resistance may continue after release from incarceration even when the person remains under the jurisdiction of the criminal justice system (Feder, 1991; Harris and Koepsell, 1996). Moreover, for many individuals, the nature and extent of their mental illness and propensity for criminal behavior place them at risk to the community. This risk is heightened if they are resistant to treatment, a fact that the treating professional must always keep in mind.

To underscore this problem, much evidence has accumulated in recent years supporting a relationship between mental illness and violence, especially among persons who are currently psychotic, do not take their medications, and are substance abusers (Monahan, 1992; Mulvey, 1994; Torrey, 1994; Hodgins and others, 1996; Marzuk, 1996; Fulwiler and others, 1997; Steadman, 1997; Swanson and others, 1997). The mental health system finds many resistant mentally ill persons extremely difficult to treat and is reluctant or unable to serve them (Jemelka, Trupin, and Chiles, 1989; Draine, Solomon, and Meyerson, 1994). The reluctance becomes even greater after these persons have committed offenses, become involved in the criminal justice system, and are referred to community agencies.

The disinclination to serve these persons extends to virtually all areas of community-based care, including therapeutic housing, social and vocational rehabilitation, and general social services (Jemelka, Trupin, and Chiles, 1989). Moreover, many mentally ill offenders are intimidating because of previous violent, fear-inspiring behavior. Treating them is very different from helping passive, formerly institutionalized patients adapt quietly to life in the community (Bachrach, Talbott, and Meyerson, 1987). Thus, community mental health professionals not only are reluctant but may also be afraid to treat offenders with mental disorders (Lamb and Weinberger, 1998). Professionals may work in treatment facilities that do not adequately provide for staff safety, do not possess the authority and leverage of the criminal justice system, and do not provide treatment interventions with adequate structure for this population.

Another important obstacle to severely mentally ill offenders' receiving outpatient treatment is that community mental health resources may be inappropriate (Knecht and others, 1996; Teplin, Abram, and McClelland, 1996). For instance, they may be expected to come to outpatient clinics, when the real need for many in this population is for outreach services where professionals come to them.

Identifying a Treatment Philosophy. To work effectively with this extremely difficult group of patients, several writers have emphasized the necessity of identifying and articulating a treatment philosophy of both theory and practice (Miraglia and Giglio, 1993; California Department of Mental Health, 1985; Lamb, Weinberger, and Gross, 1988a). This philosophy, as already mentioned, should strike a balance between individual rights and public safety and use treatment services that take both into account (Heilbrun and Griffin, 1998). A reality-based treatment philosophy is needed, one that includes clear treatment goals, with attention paid to goals expressed by the patient; a close liaison with the court or other criminal justice agency monitoring the patient, including access to each patient's database from the criminal justice and mental health systems; and an emphasis on structure and supervision.

The philosophy should also include the need for treatment staff who are comfortable using authority and setting limits, emphasis on the management of violence and recognition of the importance of psychoactive medication, and incorporation of the principles of case management. Appropriately supportive and structured living arrangements should also be a focus, with an emphasis on patients' ability to handle transition. Finally, the philosophy should recognize the role of family members and significant others in the treatment of patients.

It is also important to emphasize the legal and ethical aspects of treating persons under the jurisdiction of the criminal justice system. Before mentally ill offenders are asked to consent to outpatient treatment, they should be apprised of all the conditions and limitations that will be imposed on them, why they will be imposed, and what will happen if they do not comply (Wack, 1993). Areas to be addressed include limits to confidentiality, with respect to both past and present treatment and criminal history, and conditions under which such information must be shared with criminal justice system personnel (Heilbrun and Griffin, 1998); supervision and monitoring by various authority figures, such as probation or parole officers, judges, therapists, and case managers; mandatory compliance with treatment and other imposed conditions; and residence in an appropriate living situation. The patient must understand that noncompliance with the terms and conditions may result in revocation of outpatient status. It is also imperative that the treatment staff understand fully the patient's legal status and conditions for community placement and agree to monitor and uphold them. Staff members must accept their role as agents of social control.

Behavioral contracting has gained many adherents (Wack, 1993; Kirschenbaum and Flanery, 1984; Meichenbaum and Turk, 1987). In a forensic setting, a behavioral contract may be developed with patients in which they are clearly informed about the treatment conditions to which they must adhere and the consequences for violating them. These conditions may include medication compliance; keeping therapy and case management appointments; refraining from alcohol and drug use, with blood and urine screening to monitor substance use; not possessing weapons; living in a specified and supportive housing situation; seeking and retaining employment; and having no contact with victims of their crimes (Heilbrun and Griffin, 1998).

Treatment Goals. Generally, forensic mental health professionals believe that community treatment of severely mentally ill offenders should focus on stabilization of the illness, enhancement of independent functioning, and maintenance of internal and external controls that prevent patients from acting violently and committing other offenses. It is hoped that patients will share these goals. Patients should at least have the goal of avoiding further involvement with the criminal justice system (Smith and Berlin, 1981). Important points for discussions between the clinician and the patient are the patient's understanding of which behaviors and symptoms are of concern, why they are of concern, what is expected of the patient by both the clinician and the supervising criminal justice agency, and how the treatment can help the patient to meet these expectations (Brelje, 1985).

Even patients with severe psychiatric symptoms may be able to understand these elements of treatment and adopt appropriate attitudes toward treatment (Monahan, 1981). Thus, a full resolution of symptoms is not always needed for treatment to be viable in a community setting. For some chronic and severely mentally ill persons, total elimination of symptoms is not a realistic goal. Rather, the primary prerequisite for safe and effective community treatment may be patients' ability to understand and accept their clinical needs and the system's legal requirements and to demonstrate compliance (Wasyliw, Cavenaugh, and Grossman, 1988).

Liaison Between Treatment Staff and the Justice System. An essential aspect of treatment is a close liaison between treatment staff and the criminal justice system, including the court, the district attorney's office, the departments of probation and parole, and the patient's counsel (Bloom, Bradford, and Kofoed, 1988). At the core of the liaison is a complete and relevant database, which is fundamental in understanding the extent of the patient's problems, determining whether outpatient treatment is appropriate for the patient, and developing a treatment plan. The database should include arrest reports, "rap sheets," hospital records, evaluations by court-appointed psychiatrists or psychologists, results of psychological testing, probation reports, and records from previous hospitalizations, outpatient treatment, and incarcerations.

A successful liaison requires open, frequent, and continuing contact between the two agencies. In addition, both must respect the other's perspective and accept that they are both working toward the same goals. Together the mental health and criminal justice systems lend their expertise in developing and modifying the most effective community treatment program for patients. Both must accept that such a program cannot be effective for certain individuals.

The Need for Structure. Usually, patients referred for mandatory outpatient treatment lack internal controls; they need external controls and structure to organize them to cope with life's demands (Buckley and Bigelow, 1992; Heilbrun and Griffin, 1993; Lamb, 1997). For instance, forensic mental health professionals generally believe that staff should insist that patients' days be structured through meaningful, therapeutic activities such as work, day treatment, and various forms of social therapy (Lamb, Weinberger, and Gross, 1988b). Another basic element of structure for this population is that treatment is mandatory and under the jurisdiction of the criminal justice system.

What effect does involuntary treatment have on severely mentally ill offenders? Compliance has been shown to increase when offenders are required to undergo involuntary treatment (Hoffman, 1990; Heilbrun and Griffin, 1998). Compliance is important because it is generally assumed that severely mentally ill offenders who do not comply with treatment present an increased risk to the community. Thus, treatment noncompliance may in and of itself result in incarceration or rehospitalization.

In many ways, the criminal justice system tends to view outpatient treatment or conditional release programs as a privilege and as provisional;

such programs are not regarded as the right of the mentally ill offender (Hafemeister and Petrila, 1994). Thus, the courts are not obliged to grant such treatment. If granted, the courts allow the state to revoke it quickly and easily. The possibility of revocation of outpatient status gives the treatment staff powerful leverage to ensure adherence to the treatment conditions.

Using Authority Comfortably. A clear conception of the clinical uses and therapeutic value of authority appears to be a cornerstone of successful community treatment for severely mentally ill offenders (Wack, 1993; Lamb, Weinberger, and Gross, 1988a; Bloom, Bradford, and Kofoed, 1988). When treatment is effective, the staff are not ambivalent about the use of authority. They are comfortable about insisting consistently and reasonably that the imposed conditions be followed, monitoring patients' compliance with prescribed psychoactive medications, and monitoring patients to detect the use of alcohol or illegal drugs. They have no problems with insisting that patients live in appropriately structured and supportive residential settings as a condition for remaining in the community. They are willing to rehospitalize patients in community facilities promptly at times of crises and are willing to recommend revocation of patients' community status and return them to the responsible criminal justice agency with the opinion that community treatment is no longer appropriate.

Encouraging staff to use their authority and resolve whatever concerns they may have about doing so is essential for effective mandated outpatient treatment. Although there is far more to such treatment than simply setting limits and conducting surveillance, mental health professionals may feel ambivalent about enforcing the essential elements of this type of treatment (Miraglia and Giglio, 1993) or may have a need to always be perceived positively by their patients. In some cases, difficulty in setting limits may indicate a lack of real caring for patients (Wack, 1993).

Management of Violence. It is important that therapy focus on high-priority issues such as the need for the patient to control impulses and inappropriate expressions of anger (Wasyliw, Cavanaugh, and Grossman, 1988). Persons whose violence is rooted in an Axis I condition often experience their violence as a frightening loss of control (Wack, 1993). Because their violent acts often occur in the context of psychosis, they tend to perceive a clinician who is not aware of their destructive potential as unable to protect them. Similarly, persons whose violence is rooted in a personality disorder need the safety of knowing that the clinician is aware of their potential for violent behavior and will act to control it. They tend to establish that knowledge by testing the clinician for limits. The clinician must be continuously alert and firm in order not to risk being perceived as uncaring and unable to protect the patient from his or her own destructiveness. Wack (1993) believes that treatment contracts that deal with expectations and consequences openly and from the beginning provide a helpful structure for working with these potentially violent patients.

Dvoskin and Steadman (1994) have pointed out that persons with severe mental illness, especially those with histories of violent behavior, generally need continuous rather than episodic care. Thus, regular monitoring is needed, especially when symptoms are absent or at a low ebb, to deal with individual and situational factors that may result in violence.

For this mentally ill population, a large number of whom have problems involving control and violence, the importance of antipsychotic medications, including the atypical antipsychotic agents, cannot be overemphasized (Harris and Rice, 1997; Buckley and others, 1997). Evidence also supports the use of other agents, such as beta blockers, carbamazepine, selective serotonin reuptake inhibitors, and lithium (Buckley and others, 1997; Corrigan, Yudofsky, and Silver, 1993). In addition, behavioral, cognitive, and psychoeducational techniques emphasizing anger management have been widely used in the treatment and management of violence (Corrigan, Yudofsky, and Silver, 1993; Maier, 1993; Anderson-Malico, 1994).

In discussing problems of noncompliance, Diamond (1983) states that a closely related issue is that of autonomy, or the need for individuals to feel free of disorder and in control of their lives. Severely mentally ill persons who have been incarcerated frequently enter outpatient treatment while still taking medication and may for the first time in years find themselves symptom free, in control of their violent impulses, and able to function in the community. After a while they may feel that they can succeed without medication; they discontinue its use, decompensate, and perhaps engage in violent behavior. For some, such an experience, more than anything a clinician may say to them, ultimately convinces them that they need to stay on medication even when asymptomatic. However, if compliance is to be ensured, some patients must live in a community facility in which each dose is dispensed by staff.

Integrating Treatment and Case Management. Solomon (1992) has identified case management as a "coordinated strategy on behalf of clients to obtain the services that they need, when they need them and for as long as they need these services" (p. 164). The integration of modern concepts of case management with clinical treatment is an important component of successful outpatient treatment for mentally ill offenders (California Department of Mental Health, 1985; Bloom and others, 1986; Dvoskin and Steadman, 1994). Almost all these patients need the basic elements of case management, which starts with the premise that each patient has a designated professional with overall responsibility for his or her care.

The case manager formulates an individualized treatment and rehabilitation plan with the patient's participation. As care progresses, the case manager monitors the patient to determine if he or she is receiving treatment, has an appropriate living situation, has adequate funds, and has access to vocational rehabilitation (Hodge and Draine, 1993). The treatment plan emphasizes helping the patient deal with practical problems of daily living. In addition, the case manager provides outreach services to the patient wherever he or she is living, whether alone, with family, in a board-and-care home, or in another residential setting.

Outreach services may take the form of assertive case management. An assertive case management program deals with patients on a frequent and long-term basis. It takes a hands-on approach that may necessitate meeting with patients on their own turf or even seeing a patient daily (Wilson, Tien, and Eaves, 1995). This form of contact and familiarity with the patient helps the case manager anticipate and prevent a significant decompensation. Low caseloads for case managers of potentially violent mentally ill persons—probably not more than ten cases—have been recommended, as has twenty-four-hour, seven-day-a-week availability (Dvoskin and Steadman, 1994). Many violent acts and arrests occur during evenings, nights, and weekends, when traditional treatment programs are closed.

Before accepting case management, some mentally ill offenders first ask, "What's in it for me?" (Dvoskin and Steadman, 1994). Patients who perceive the case manager as mainly an agent of the criminal justice system, whose primary intention is to make them toe the line, will be less likely to form a positive relationship with a case manager. They may be guarded and defensive in their interactions. Patients may be less inclined to be candid and may feel a need to portray themselves in a good light, even though they have problems for which they need help. Therefore, patients must see the case manager as their advocate to further their treatment and rehabilitation, particularly when agencies in the criminal justice system are simultaneously dealing with them in more coercive or authoritarian ways.

Dvoskin and Steadman (1994) discuss some of the stress and problems case managers experience. They may feel, with some justification, that they are in personal danger if they work with mentally ill offenders who have been violent in the past or if their work requires visits to high-crime areas, where many persons with serious mental illness live. Additional problems may include unusual working hours, which may disrupt their family and social relationships, and lack of upward career mobility. Finally, forensic case managers may feel mixed loyalties to their clients and the criminal justice system in terms of role contradictions (Solomon and Draine, 1995).

Therapeutic Living Arrangements. Survival in the community for the great majority of offenders with serious mental illness appears to depend on an appropriately supportive and structured living arrangement (Lamb, Weinberger, and Gross, 1988a). Such an arrangement can often be provided by family members. However, in many cases, the kind and degree of structure the patient needs can be found only in a living arrangement outside the family home, with a high staff-patient ratio, dispensing of medication by staff, enforcement of curfews, and therapeutic activities that structure most of the patient's day.

Some patients need a great deal of structure and supervision in their housing situation, others need only a minimal amount, and most fall somewhere in between. How much structure does a patient need? The treatment staff member assigned to the patient or the patient's case manager must decide whether a particular living arrangement has the appropriate amount of structure to meet the patient's needs. However, it is necessary to first discuss the suggested living arrangement with the responsible agent in the criminal justice system and obtain his or her approval.

A consideration for all patients who move from a closed or locked setting such as a forensic hospital, jail, or prison is the patient's ability to handle transition (Shively and Petrich, 1985; Derks, Blankstein, and Hendrickx, 1993; Nuehring and Raybin, 1986). It is generally not advisable for persons who have been hospitalized or incarcerated for a long time to be placed in the community in a living situation with little or no structure. Such individuals are frequently unable to cope with the immediate stress and demands of these arrangements, and they either decompensate or commit subsequent offenses.

Therefore, it is helpful to release many severely mentally ill offenders to graduated lower levels of structure—for example, from prison or a forensic hospital to a locked community facility to a halfway house and, when they are ready, to family or independent living. In the graduated release process, close attention must be paid to patients' coping skills and need for monitoring. A brief hospital stay may be necessary when patients decompensate under stress.

Working with the Family. The role of family members or significant others can be critical in the treatment of mentally ill offenders (Lamb and Weinberger, 1998). The treatment team should determine whether these individuals were the victims of the patient's aggression and whether they have maintained contact with the patient. The team should also learn whether other social support systems are available while the patient resides in the community. Social support can be an extremely important part of community treatment for mentally ill offenders (Wasyliw, Cavanaugh, and Grossman, 1988; Jacoby and Kozie-Peak, 1997). Assessing problems that may develop between the patient and family members or significant others is essential if contact between them is anticipated.

Another important consideration is the family members' needs for guidance and support, especially when they have been victimized by the patient. Clinicians should help them understand the patient's mental condition, teaching them to recognize symptoms of decompensation, demonstrating methods for self-protection, and explaining the patient's current legal situation (Lamb and Weinberger, 1998; Lefley, 1987; McFarland and others, 1990; Nedopil and Banzer, 1996).

Moreover, family members should be involved in support groups to help them during crises; in self-help programs, they can benefit from the experience of other families in similar situations (Hylton, 1995).

Pitfalls. Mental health professionals must understand their potential liability for the actions of their patients who are on community status (Hafemeister and Petrila, 1994; Miller and others, 1988). They need to be aware that in some states, courts have imposed on therapists a duty of care that extends to foreseeability of harm. Moreover, the litigious nature of our society adds further pressures and risks. Treating clinicians may be held accountable for patients' suicides, assaults, homicides, and other crimes, even when treatment was mandated, sound, and met the professional community's standards of care. In both public agencies and private practice, malpractice insurance coverage must be adequate so that clinicians feel comfortable, personally and professionally, in undertaking the treatment of severely mentally ill offenders.

Another important concern of clinicians involved in the community treatment of mentally ill offenders—especially sex offenders and other persons who have committed high-profile crimes—is the possibility of notoriety and unfavorable publicity. Clinicians may fear that if patients commit further sensational crimes, their professional reputation will suffer.

Rice and Harris (1997) point out the conflicting pressures on professionals attempting to treat mentally ill offenders. The pressures may be unrelated to objective considerations about what is best for the patient and the treatment. On the one hand, a variety of formal and informal complaints and lawsuits may be lodged by patients about their detained (locked) status; they may argue that they no longer pose a danger to society and are ready for community rehabilitation. For such reasons, some mentally ill offenders may be inappropriately released to community treatment. On the other hand, if a mentally ill offender in community treatment commits a high-profile crime, the agency and the clinician may have to deal with an understandably angry community and devote much time and energy to defending themselves and perhaps preparing for litigation.

Furthermore, it must be recognized that not all mentally ill offenders can be treated effectively in the community. Tellefson and others (1992) emphasize the importance of identifying high-risk patients so that scarce treatment resources are used for those most likely to succeed and least likely to incur the high costs of hospitalization and rearrest for exacerbations of illness or aggressive behavior.

Conclusion

Creating a successful treatment program for severely mentally ill offenders is a difficult task that demands the input and cooperation of professionals who are knowledgeable and accepting of the tenets of both the criminal justice system and mental health treatment. The terms and conditions for community outpatient treatment imposed by the criminal justice system should not be developed in a vacuum. It is strongly recommended that mental health professionals familiar with forensic patients and issues be consulted from the beginning. That is, forensic clinicians should have input into determining under what conditions and when a patient is ready for outpatient status. If such conditions exist and if they ensure that the patient does not pose a threat of harm, community treatment should be instituted.

As mentally ill offenders are treated in the community, it is hoped that a close liaison develops between mental health treatment staff and criminal justice system personnel to assess patients' progress and needs. With frequent consultation and respect between these two professional groups, a trusting relationship can be fostered that will ultimately benefit both patients and the community.

References

Anderson-Malico, R. "Anger Management Using Cognitive Group Therapy." *Perspectives in Psychiatric Care, 30,* 1994, 17–20.

Bachrach, L. L., Talbott, J. A., and Meyerson, A. T. "The Chronic Psychiatric Patient as a 'Difficult' Patient: A Conceptual Analysis." In A. T. Meyerson (ed.), *Barriers to Treating the Chronic Mentally Ill.* New Directions for Mental Health Services, no. 33. San Francisco: Jossey-Bass, 1987.

Bloom, J. D., Bradford, J. M., and Kofoed, L. "An Overview of Psychiatric Treatment Approaches to Three Offender Groups." *Hospital and Community Psychiatry,* 1988, *39,* 151–158.

Bloom, J. D., and others. "Evaluation and Treatment of Insanity Acquittees in the Community." *Bulletin of the American Academy of Psychiatry and the Law,* 1986, *14,* 231–244.

Borzecki, M. A., and Wormith, J. S. "The Criminalization of Psychiatrically Ill People: A Review with a Canadian Perspective." *Psychiatric Journal of the University of Ottawa,* 1985, *10,* 241–247.

Brelje, T. B. "Problems of Treatment of NGRIs in an Inpatient Mental Health System." Paper presented at a meeting of the Illinois Association of Community Mental Health Agencies, Chicago, 1985.

Buckley, P. F., and others. "Aggression and Schizophrenia: Efficacy of Risperidone." *Journal of the American Academy of Psychiatry and the Law,* 1997, *25,* 173–181.

Buckley, R., and Bigelow, D. A. "The Multi-Service Network: Reaching the Unserved Multi-Problem Individual." *Community Mental Health Journal,* 1992, *28,* 43–50.

Bullard, H. "Management of Violent Patients." In J. Shepherd (ed.), *Violence in Health Care: A Practical Guide to Coping with Violence and Caring for Victims.* New York: Oxford University Press, 1994.

California Department of Mental Health. *California Department of Mental Health Conditional Release Program for the Judicially Committed.* Sacramento: California Department of Mental Health, 1985.

Cohen, A., and Eastman, N. "Needs Assessment for Mentally Disordered Offenders and Others Requiring Similar Services." *British Journal of Psychiatry,* 1997, *171,* 412–416.

Corrigan, P. W., Yudofsky, S. C., and Silver, J. M. "Pharmacological and Behavioral Treatments for Aggressive Psychiatric Inpatients." *Hospital and Community Psychiatry,* 1993, *44,* 125–133.

Derks, F.C.H., Blankstein, J. H., and Hendrickx, J.J.P. "Treatment and Security: The Dual Nature of Forensic Psychiatry." *International Journal of Law and Psychiatry,* 1993, *16,* 217–240.

Diamond, R. J. "Enhancing Medication Use in Schizophrenic Patients." *Journal of Clinical Psychiatry,* 1983, *44,* 7–14.

Draine, J., Solomon, P., and Meyerson, A. "Predictors of Reincarceration Among Patients Who Received Psychiatric Services in Jail." *Hospital and Community Psychiatry,* 1994, *45,* 163–167.

Dvoskin, J. A., and Steadman, H. J. "Using Intensive Case Management to Reduce Violence by Mentally Ill Persons in the Community." *Hospital and Community Psychiatry,* 1994, *45,* 679–684.

Feder, L. "A Comparison of the Community Adjustment of Mentally Ill Offenders with Those from the General Prison Population: An 18-Month Follow Up." *Law and Human Behavior,* 1991, *15,* 477–493.

Fulwiler, C., and others. "Early-Onset Substance Abuse and Community Violence by Outpatients with Chronic Mental Illness." *Psychiatric Services,* 1997, *48,* 1181–1185.

Griffin, P. A., Steadman, H. J., and Heilbrun, K. "Designing Conditional Release Systems for Insanity Acquittees." *Journal of Mental Health Administration,* 1991, *18,* 231–241.

Hafemeister, T. L., and Petrila, J. "Treating the Mentally Disordered Offender: Society's Uncertain, Conflicted, and Changing Views." *Florida State University Law Review,* 1994, *21,* 729–871.

Harris, G. T., and Rice, M. E. "Risk Appraisal and Management of Violent Behavior." *Psychiatric Services,* 1997, *48,* 1168–1176.

Harris, V., and Koepsell, T. D. "Criminal Recidivism in Mentally Ill Offenders: A Pilot Study." *Bulletin of the American Academy of Psychiatry and the Law,* 1996, *24,* 177–186.

Heilbrun, K., and Griffin, P. A. "Community-Based Forensic Treatment of Insanity Acquittees." *International Journal of Law and Psychiatry,* 1993, *16,* 133–150.

Heilbrun, K., and Griffin, P. A. "Community-Based Forensic Treatment." In R. M. Wettstein (ed.), *Treatment of Offenders with Mental Disorders.* New York: Guilford Press, 1998.

Hodge, M., and Draine, J. "Development of Support Through Case Management Services." In R. Flexer and P. Solomon (eds.), *Psychiatric Rehabilitation in Practice.* New York: Andover Medical, 1993.

Hodgins, S., and others. "Mental Disorder and Crime: Evidence from a Danish Birth Cohort." *Archives of General Psychiatry,* 1996, *53,* 489–496.

Hoffman, B. F. "The Criminalization of the Mentally Ill." *Canadian Journal of Psychiatry,* 1990, *35,* 166–169.

Hylton, J. H. "Care or Control: Health or Criminal Justice Options for the Long-Term Seriously Mentally Ill in a Canadian Province." *International Journal of Law and Psychiatry,* 1995, *18,* 45–59.

Jacoby, J. E., and Kozie-Peak, B. "The Benefits of Social Support for Mentally Ill Offenders: Prison-to-Community Transitions." *Behavioral Sciences and the Law,* 1997, *15,* 483–501.

Jemelka, R. P., Trupin, E., and Chiles, J. A. "The Mentally Ill in Prison: A Review." *Hospital and Community Psychiatry,* 1989, *40,* 481–491.

Kirschenbaum, D. S., and Flanery, R. C. "Toward a Psychology of Behavioral Contracting." *Clinical Psychology Review,* 1984, *4,* 597–618.

Knecht, G., and others. "Outpatient Treatment of Mentally Disordered Offenders in Austria." *International Journal of Law and Psychiatry,* 1996, *19,* 87–91.

Laberge, D., and Morin, D. "The Overuse of Criminal Justice Dispositions: Failure of Diversionary Policies in the Management of Mental Health Problems." *International Journal of Law and Psychiatry,* 1995, *18,* 389–414.

Lamb, H. R. "Incompetency to Stand Trial: Appropriateness and Outcome." *Archives of General Psychiatry,* 1987, *44,* 754–758.

Lamb, H. R. "The New State Mental Hospitals in the Community." *Psychiatric Services,* 1997, *48,* 1307–1310.

Lamb, H. R., and Weinberger, L. E. "Persons with Severe Mental Illness in Jails and Prisons: A Review." *Psychiatric Services,* 1998, *4,* 483–492.

Lamb, H. R., Weinberger, L. E., and Gross, B. H. "Court-Mandated Outpatient Treatment for Insanity Acquittees: Clinical Philosophy and Implementation." *Hospital and Community Psychiatry,* 1988a, *39,* 1080–1084.

Lamb, H. R., Weinberger, L. E., and Gross, B. H. "Court-Mandated Community Outpatient Treatment for Persons Found Not Guilty by Reason of Insanity: A Five-Year Follow-Up." *American Journal of Psychiatry,* 1988b, *145,* 450–456.

Lefley, H. P. "Aging Parents as Caregivers of Mentally Ill Adult Children: An Emerging Social Problem." *Hospital and Community Psychiatry,* 1987, *38,* 1063–1070.

Maier, G. J. "Management Approaches for the Repetitively Aggressive Patient." In W. H. Sledge and A. Tasman (eds.), *Clinical Challenges in Psychiatry*. Washington, D.C.: American Psychiatric Press, 1993.

Marzuk, P. M. "Violence, Crime, and Mental Illness: How Strong a Link?" *Archives of General Psychiatry*, 1996, 53, 481–486.

McFarland, B. H., and others. "Family Members' Opinions About Civil Commitment." *Hospital and Community Psychiatry*, 1990, 41, 537–540.

Meichenbaum, D., and Turk, D. *Facilitating Treatment Adherence: A Practitioner's Guidebook*. New York: Plenum, 1987.

Miller, R. D., and others. "Emerging Problems for Staff Associated with the Release of Potentially Dangerous Forensic Patients." *Bulletin of the American Academy of Psychiatry and the Law*, 1988, 16, 309–320.

Miraglia, R. P., and Giglio, C. A. "Refining an Aftercare Program for New York State's Outpatient Insanity Acquittees." *Psychiatric Quarterly*, 1993, 64, 215–234.

Monahan, J. *Predicting Violent Behavior: An Assessment of Clinical Techniques*. Thousand Oaks, Calif.: Sage, 1981.

Monahan, J. "Mental Disorder and Violent Behavior: Perceptions and Evidence." *American Psychologist*, 1992, 47, 511–521.

Morris, G. H. "Placed in Purgatory: Conditional Release of Insanity Acquittees." *Arizona Law Review*, 1997, 39, 1061–1114.

Mulvey, E. P. "Assessing the Evidence of a Link Between Mental Illness and Violence." *Hospital and Community Psychiatry*, 1994, 45, 663–668.

Nedopil, N., and Banzer, K. "Outpatient Treatment of Forensic Patients in Germany: Current Structure and Future Developments." *International Journal of Law and Psychiatry*, 1996, 19, 75–79.

Nuehring, E. M., and Raybin, L. "Mentally Ill Offenders in Community Based Programs: Attitudes of Service Providers." *Journal of Offender Counseling, Services, and Rehabilitation*, 1986, 11, 19–37.

Rice, M. E., and Harris, G. T. "The Treatment of Mentally Disordered Offenders." *Psychology, Public Policy, and Law*, 1997, 3, 126–183.

Robertson, G., Pearson, R., and Gibb, R. "The Entry of Mentally Disordered People to the Criminal Justice System." *British Journal of Psychiatry*, 1996, 169, 172–180.

Shively, D., and Petrich, J. "Correctional Mental Health." *Psychiatric Clinics of North America*, 1985, 8, 537–550.

Smith, A. B., and Berlin, L. *Treating the Criminal Offender*. Upper Saddle River, N.J.: Prentice-Hall, 1981.

Solomon, P. "The Efficacy of Case Management Services for Severely Mentally Disabled Clients." *Community Mental Health Journal*, 1992, 28, 163–180.

Solomon, P., and Draine, J. "Jail Recidivism in a Forensic Case Management Program." *Health and Social Work*, 1995, 20, 167–173.

Steadman, H. J. "Risk Factors for Community Violence Among Acute Psychiatric Inpatients: The MacArthur Risk Assessment Project." Paper presented at the annual meeting of the American Psychiatric Association, San Diego, May 17–22, 1997.

Swanson, J., and others. "Violence and Severe Mental Disorder in Clinical and Community Populations: The Effects of Psychotic Symptoms, Comorbidity, and Lack of Treatment." *Psychiatry*, 1997, 60, 1–22.

Tellefsen, C., and others. "Predicting Success on Conditional Release for Insanity Acquittees: Regionalized Versus Nonregionalized Hospital Patients." *Bulletin of the American Academy of Psychiatry and the Law*, 1992, 20, 87–100.

Teplin, L. A., Abram, K. M., and McClelland, G. M. "Prevalence of Psychiatric Disorders Among Incarcerated Women." *Archives of General Psychiatry*, 1996, 53, 505–512.

Torrey, E. F. "Violent Behavior by Individuals with Serious Mental Illness." *Hospital and Community Psychiatry*, 1994, 45, 653–662.

Wack, R. C. "The Ongoing Risk Assessment in the Treatment of Forensic Patients on Conditional Release Status." *Psychiatric Quarterly*, 1993, 6, 275–293.

Wasyliw, O. E., Cavanaugh, J. L., and Grossman, L. S. "Clinical Considerations in the Community Treatment of Mentally Disordered Offenders." *International Journal of Law and Psychiatry*, 1988, 11, 371–380.

Wilson, D., Tien, G., and Eaves, D. "Increasing the Community Tenure of Mentally Disordered Offenders: An Assertive Case Management Program." *International Journal of Law and Psychiatry*, 1995, 18, 61–69.

H. RICHARD LAMB *is professor of psychiatry and the behavioral sciences at Keck School of Medicine, University of Southern California, in Los Angeles.*

LINDA E. WEINBERGER *is professor of clinical psychiatry and chief psychologist at the Institute of Psychiatry, Law, and Behavioral Sciences at Keck School of Medicine, University of Southern California, in Los Angeles.*

BRUCE H. GROSS *is associate professor of psychiatry and director of the Institute of Psychiatry, Law, and Behavioral Sciences at Keck School of Medicine, University of Southern California, in Los Angeles.*

5

Outreach emergency teams comprising police officers and mental health professionals can help to avoid criminalization of the mentally ill.

Outcome for Psychiatric Emergency Patients Seen by an Outreach Police–Mental Health Team

H. Richard Lamb, Roderick Shaner, Diana M. Elliott, Walter J. DeCuir Jr., James T. Foltz

Emergency psychiatric outreach to mentally ill persons, combined with access to hospital-based psychiatric services, has been shown to be a needed mental health resource (Cohen, 1991; Zealberg and others, 1992; Gillig, Dumaine, and Hillard, 1990). Severely mentally ill persons are at risk of criminalization, defined as inappropriate diversion to the criminal justice system, and a certain proportion of mentally ill persons in crisis may become violent.

Considerable evidence points to the criminalization of mentally ill persons; that is, large numbers of persons with severe mental illness who have committed minor crimes are taken to jails instead of to hospitals or other psychiatric treatment facilities (Torrey and others, 1993; Lamb, 1994; Lamb and Grant, 1982; Lamb and others, 1984). Most such persons should be diverted to the mental health system. Criminalization has been attributed to lack of adequate psychiatric resources, a revolving-door phenomenon in hospital emergency rooms and inpatient services (Lamb and Shaner, 1993; Lamb, Sorkin, and Zusman, 1981), and civil-libertarian constraints on involuntary psychiatric treatment (Lamb and Grant, 1982).

Another possible reason for criminalization is that the initial contact with many severely disturbed persons in the community is made by the police, who may not always recognize a need for—or have access to—emergency psychiatric resources. Clearly, mental health expertise is needed at this point.

The police are often the first to respond to emergencies involving persons with severe psychiatric disturbances (Zealberg and others, 1992). Data

Source: Lamb, H. R., Shaner, R., Elliott, D. M., DeCuir Jr., W. J., and Foltz, J. T. "Outcome for Psychiatric Emergency Patients Seen by an Outreach Police–Mental Health Team." *Psychiatric Services*, 1995, 46 (12), 1267–1271. Reprinted by permission.

from New York State (Way, Evans, and Banks, 1993) and Los Angeles (Morrell, 1989) have shown that at least 30 percent of persons seen in psychiatric emergency rooms are brought there by the police. Other studies have indicated that patients brought by the police are more psychiatrically disturbed, more likely to be hospitalized, more dangerous to others, and more gravely disabled than those not brought by the police (Watson, Segal, and Newhill, 1993; McNiel and others, 1991; Sales, 1991).

Generally, the potential for violence underlies most situations in which individuals present as psychiatric emergencies (Ellison, Hughes, and White, 1989; McNiel and Binder, 1987; Beck, White, and Gage, 1991). A growing body of evidence also suggests the existence of a subgroup of seriously mentally ill persons who are significantly more dangerous than the general population (Torrey, 1994; Mulvey, 1994). This subgroup poses a serious challenge. It has been observed that emergency psychiatric outreach teams comprising only mental health professionals are not able to cope with serious physical violence or the threat of it (Gillig, Dumaine, and Hillard, 1990; Zealberg, Santos, and Fisher, 1993). Thus, there are pressing needs for proficiency in the management of violence and for mental health expertise in field situations where psychiatrically ill persons are first encountered (Gillig and others, 1990).

This chapter describes a study and six-month follow-up of 101 consecutive referrals to an outreach team that included both a specially trained police officer and a mental health professional. We hypothesized that such a team would be able to make a comprehensive assessment and appropriate disposition for all psychiatric emergencies in the field, even for persons who are violent or potentially violent. We also hypothesized that if the team evaluated mentally ill people in the field, fewer would be inappropriately placed in the criminal justice system.

The Emergency Outreach Team

The need for mental health expertise in police field situations was recognized in Los Angeles in 1985 with the formation of a mental evaluation unit in the Los Angeles Police Department. When officers in the field encounter someone they believe is mentally ill, they bring the subject to the mental evaluation unit, located in the police administration building in downtown Los Angeles, for screening. The screening is done by unit police officers specifically trained in the identification, assessment, and referral of mentally ill citizens.

The mental evaluation unit assesses more than four thousand persons a year and receives more than fifty-four thousand calls for consultation and other services annually. Most mentally ill persons who normally would have been arrested for low-grade misdemeanors have been diverted to more appropriate resources; dispositions other than jail or hospital have been found for many of them. Those who are taken to psychiatric emergency rooms are generally found by emergency room physicians to be appropriate referrals. The mental evaluation unit also provides telephone consultation to officers in the field and training to officers in various police stations.

In spite of the effectiveness of the mental evaluation unit, some problems remained intractable. Large numbers of mentally ill persons, often those who were violent or threatening, continued to enter local jails. Police officers had difficulty gaining access to emergency psychiatric resources. Mobile teams of mental health professionals had limited ability to respond to situations that had the potential for violence.

Beginning in 1991, the Los Angeles County Department of Mental Health (with strong support from the Los Angeles County Board of Supervisors) and the Los Angeles Police Department collaborated to refine their response to incidents involving mentally ill persons in crisis. The result was the development of the Systemwide Mental Assessment Response Team (SMART), a pilot program in which an outreach team comprising both a police officer with special training and a mental health professional is available on each police watch to respond to emergencies in the community. The team began operations in January 1993.

The total team consists of four police officers, a detective who supervises them, four mental health clinicians, and one mental health supervisor. All mental health personnel are funded by the Los Angeles County Department of Mental Health. The clinicians are psychiatric nurses or psychiatric technicians, and the supervisor is a licensed clinical social worker. In order to develop a team identity and a uniform approach, all team members received an initial eighty hours of instruction, as well as ongoing monthly training in crisis intervention, mental illness, first aid, weaponless self-defense, forensic issues, tactical training, community concerns, networking, and law enforcement and mental health policy and procedures.

The team is deployed seven days a week, sixteen hours a day. At least one mental health professional and one specially trained officer are on duty on each watch. Incidents reported to the police department's mental evaluation unit are referred to the team at the unit watch commander's discretion, based on the watch commander's judgment of whether mental health issues may be involved. The team travels by police vehicle to the site of the incident.

The team evaluates the disturbed person and the situation on site and makes a decision about disposition of the individual; dispositions include taking the person to a hospital psychiatric emergency room, providing a referral to outpatient or other community resources, or no services. During the pilot program, the team responded to five inner-city areas of the department's eighteen geographic areas, and expansion to other areas was planned.

Methods

The 101 consecutive referrals to SMART between September 13, 1993, and October 30, 1993, constituted the study sample. Data on demographic characteristics, clinical history, arrest history, previous violent behavior, and similar variables were drawn from the team records, which were reviewed by the authors. Team records for each case include written summaries by both the mental health professional and the police officer, as well as the subject's criminal record, if any, which the team routinely obtains from the Network Communications System (NECS) Criminal Justice Computer System. The team also routinely searches the computerized management information system of the Los Angeles County Department of Mental Health to obtain additional history.

Follow-up data are collected on all referrals, on an ongoing basis, for program evaluation. In this study, we tried to determine the subjects' follow-up status during the six months after referral to the team. Specifically, we were interested in information on hospitalizations, arrests, acts of violence, mental health treatment, and living situation. The records of all subjects were again checked through the NECS Criminal Justice Computer System and the department of mental health's management information system. Follow-up information was also obtained from family members, friends, landlords, mental health providers, and other available persons and from repeat evaluations; by the end of the follow-up period, 11 of the 101 subjects had been seen again one or more times by the team.

At six-month follow-up, the whereabouts and status of fifteen referrals were unknown. One referral had died in the hospital to which he was taken in the index episode. Thus, the follow-up group numbered eighty-five.

Chi-square analysis, with correction for continuity, was used to determine whether significant relationships existed between study variables such as history of arrest, history of serious violence against persons, previous psychiatric hospitalization, and presence of major psychopathology. The variables were dichotomized as the presence or absence of such conditions.

Results

Demographic and Clinical Characteristics at Referral. Sixty of the 101 referrals were male, and forty-one were female. Their mean ±SD age was 39±12.3 years, with a range of 19 to 74 years; the median age was 37. Seventy-one were single, fourteen were married, and sixteen were separated, divorced, or widowed. Thirty-three were black; forty-five, Caucasian; nineteen, Hispanic; and four, Asian. Forty-nine were receiving Supplemental Security Income; only eight were currently employed. Thirty-one were homeless.

On the basis of their clinical presentation, 70 of the 101 subjects were considered to have major psychopathology, defined as at least two severe overt psychiatric symptoms such as delusions, hallucinations, and disorganized thinking. Sixty-three of the subjects were known to have had a history of violence against persons. Sixty had an arrest history, and 46 had been arrested on charges of violence against persons. Seventy-nine were known to have had previous psychiatric hospitalizations. Sixty-three of the referrals were known to be poorly compliant with prescribed medications. Sixty-six were known to be serious substance abusers.

Twenty of the 101 subjects were overtly violent when seen by the team, and 29 others exhibited threatening behavior. Seventy-two manifested bizarre or disorganized behavior, 8 had made suicide attempts, 19 were threatening suicide, and 15 were engaged in self-endangering behavior. Current use of drugs and alcohol was clearly a factor in the presenting situation in 19 of the cases.

When possible, psychiatric diagnoses were obtained from the records of facilities that had been able to make an extended evaluation; almost all of the diagnoses were based on such extended evaluation. Otherwise, the diagnoses of the team were used. The largest number of referrals, 34, were diagnosed as having schizophrenia; 15, schizoaffective disorder; 14, bipolar disorder; 13, major depression without psychosis; 6, major depression with psychotic features; 6, psychosis not otherwise specified; 6, substance-induced disorders; 2, dementia; and 5, other disorders.

Disposition. Sixty-nine of the subjects were placed on involuntary seventy-two-hour holds. Eighty were taken to hospitals: 48 to county hospitals, 24 to private hospitals under Medicaid, 7 to private hospitals under private insurance, and 1 to a Veterans Administration hospital. Of the 80 taken to hospitals, 65 were involuntarily admitted, and 7 were not admitted; thus, 73 were actually hospitalized.

Only 2 of the 101 subjects were taken to jail. Twenty-six subjects were not jailed or hospitalized, including the 7 taken to hospitals but not admitted; of those 26 subjects, 11 were given outpatient referrals, 6 were referred to other community resources, 6 refused any referral, and 3 were not felt to need referrals.

Six-Month Follow-Up. Of the eighty-five referrals for whom six-month follow-up could be completed, twenty subjects (24 percent) were arrested during this period, ten of them (12 percent) for crimes of violence. During the six months, thirty-six subjects (42 percent) were hospitalized (this total excludes hospitalizations resulting from the index referral to the team), and nineteen (22 percent) committed acts of violence. At the end of the six months, thirty-three subjects (39 percent) were in outpatient mental health treatment, ten (12 percent) were in intermediate or long-term locked facilities, thirteen (15 percent) were placed on a mental health conservatorship, and nine (11 percent) were homeless.

Analysis of the data revealed some significant relationships. As Table 5.1 shows, history of serious violence against persons was significantly related to presence of major psychopathology ($\chi^2 = 6.76$, df = 1, $p \geq (.01)$) and to previous psychiatric hospitalization ($\chi^2 = 4.42$, df = 1, $p \leq .04$).

Discussion

General Considerations. The study subjects clearly presented a formidable challenge for emergency psychiatric evaluation and management in the field. The 101 referrals manifested a high incidence of overt major psychopathology, history of serious violence against others, history of criminal

Table 5.1. Relationship Between History of Serious Violence Against Persons, Presence of Major Psychopathology, and Previous Psychiatric Hospitalization Among 101 Psychiatric Emergency Patients Evaluated by a Police–Mental Health Outreach Team

| | Serious Violence Against Persons | | |
	Yes	No	Total
Major pathology[a]			
Yes	50	13	63
No	20	18	38
Total	70	31	101
Previous hospitalization[b]			
Yes	54	9	63
No	25	13	38
Total	79	22	101

[a]$\chi^2 = 6.76$ (corrected for continuity), df $= 1$, $p \le .01$.
[b]$\chi^2 = 4.42$ (corrected for continuity), df $= 1$, $p \le .04$.

arrest including arrest on charges of violence toward others, previous psychiatric hospitalizations, poor compliance with prescribed antipsychotic medications, and serious substance abuse.

Remarkably, only 2 percent of the group were taken to jail. A major contemporary social problem is the criminalization of chronically and severely mentally ill persons, or their placement in the criminal justice system for minor crimes instead of in the mental health system. Because of the use of well-trained teams consisting of a mental health professional and a police officer, these subjects were not criminalized, even though they came from a population at high risk for criminalization.

Almost all the subjects were first referred to the police, who then referred them to the team, thus automatically bringing mental health expertise into a field situation at an early stage. However, because a large proportion of the group was violent or potentially violent, mental health professionals would have had more difficulty without police assistance. Moreover, the team provided a way for violent psychiatric patients to be handled expeditiously and humanely.

The study group's history, characteristics, and presenting behaviors resemble those of psychiatric emergency patients, as reported in several studies, for whom inpatient treatment was recommended (Way, Evans, and Banks, 1992; McNiel and others, 1992; Segal and others, 1988). Thus, it is not surprising that 68 percent were placed on involuntary seventy-two-hour holds. However, 19 percent of the subjects were not taken to hospitals or jails; in these cases, the work of the team was evaluation and crisis intervention.

The percentages of the sample with prior arrests (59 percent) and prior arrests for crimes of violence (46 percent) are remarkably high, even considering that the referrals were all seen in an inner-city area. These data indicate the value of access to computerized criminal justice records and are consistent with findings of a similar study of police referral to psychiatric emergency services (Watson, Segal, and Newhill, 1993). The high percentage of known substance abuse is also consistent with emergency room studies (Barbee and others, 1989; Szuster, Schanbacher, and McCann, 1990; Elangovan and others, 1993; Galanter, Castaneda, and Ferman, 1988).

In the six-month follow-up period, 24 percent of the eighty-five subjects in the follow-up were arrested, 12 percent for crimes of violence. Although we do not have data to explain this finding, we can speculate that a team incorporating both law enforcement and mental health personnel more successfully avoids criminalization. For instance, most of the subjects were subsequently encountered in the field by police officers not accompanied by mental health professionals.

That 42 percent of the follow-up group were rehospitalized and 22 percent committed acts of violence during the six-month follow-up would indicate that most of them were not successfully treated during that period. On the other hand, 39 percent were in outpatient mental health treatment, 12 percent were in intermediate or long-term locked facilities, and 15 percent had been placed on mental health conservatorship, indicating that many of the group's mental health needs had been met. Still another positive finding was that only 11 percent were homeless at follow-up, compared with 31 percent at referral to the team. That almost a third of the subjects were initially homeless is consistent with findings that a large proportion of homeless persons are severely mentally ill (Lamb, 1984; Baum and Burnes, 1993).

The study found a strong relationship between presence of overt major psychopathology and a history of serious violence against persons, which is evidence that in the evaluation and disposition of seriously mentally ill people in crisis in the community, personnel such as police officers with special training and expertise in the humane management of violence are needed. The relationship between a history of serious violence against persons and previous psychiatric hospitalizations provides further evidence.

Treatment Issues. The team benefits from shared access to mental health and criminal justice information. The police officer on the team has access to county mental health records of the referrals, and the mental health professional has access to criminal justice data on the referrals' arrest records, warrants, prior police contacts for psychiatric problems, and weapon ownership; both kinds of information are useful for understanding the subject in an emergency situation and making a disposition decision. Confidentiality must be respected; law enforcement and mental health personnel may not share information from the other system's records with colleagues outside the team, and information in team records may not be revealed to the police department or other law enforcement agencies.

In this new endeavor, the police officer provides security, transportation, law enforcement field resources, and the knowledge of how to deal with violence effectively and humanely. The mental health professional provides knowledge about mental illness, training in diagnosis and crisis evaluation, and experience in relating to psychiatric patients. Also invaluable is the mental health professional's familiarity with mental health resources and their admission criteria. The teams save badly needed county hospital and jail bed space; when possible, they can divert the referral to a private hospital, substance abuse center, or outpatient mental health program.

The team not only enhances the effectiveness of officers in the field but also can be a more effective alternative to the mobile psychiatric response teams deployed by many public and private mental health agencies. These mobile teams, staffed only by mental health personnel, are less prepared to respond alone to calls that may involve a potentially violent person (Gillig, Dumaine, and Hillard, 1990; Zealberg, Santos, and Fisher, 1993). Without law enforcement involvement, the mental health condition of many patients in crisis in the community may further deteriorate. Moreover, psychiatric mobile response teams, unlike the police, may not have twenty-four-hour access to backup transportation and personnel.

Establishing such teams is not without problems. For instance, mental health professionals begin with relatively little awareness of law enforcement procedures and policies. However, with time and training, they become more familiar and comfortable with public safety issues. Similarly, the police officers begin with relatively little formal knowledge and training about psychiatric problems, although they possess a keen street sense that is a valuable resource for the team. With time and training, the officers develop a good understanding of mental health issues and become able to participate effectively in referral decisions. The importance of training, both initial and ongoing, cannot be overemphasized.

Conclusion

We have shown that psychiatric emergency teams consisting of police officers and mental health professionals are able to deal with psychiatric emergencies in the field, even with a population characterized by acute and chronic severe mental illness, a high potential for violence, a high incidence of serious substance abuse, and long histories with both the criminal justice and the mental health systems.

The teams provide a response that combines the specialized knowledge and expertise of both law enforcement and mental health professionals. They can greatly increase the number of mentally ill persons who are given appropriate access to the mental health system rather than inappropriately diverted to the criminal justice system. They facilitate the expeditious and humane handling of psychiatric patients who are violent. We believe that the use of such teams is an advance in the evaluation, management, and disposition of psychiatric emergencies in the field.

References

Barbee, J. G., and others. "Alcohol and Substance Abuse Among Schizophrenic Patients Presenting to an Emergency Psychiatric Service." *Journal of Nervous and Mental Disease*, 1989, *177*, 400–407.

Baum, A. S., and Burnes, D. W. *A Nation in Denial: The Truth About Homelessness.* Boulder, Colo.: Westview Press, 1993.

Beck, J. C., White, K. A., and Gage, B. "Emergency Psychiatric Assessment of Violence." *American Journal of Psychiatry*, 1991, *148*, 1562–1565.

Cohen, N. L. (ed.). *Psychiatric Outreach to the Mentally Ill.* New Directions for Mental Health Services, no. 52. San Francisco: Jossey-Bass, 1991.

Elangovan, N., and others. "Substance Abuse Among Patients Presenting at an Inner-City Psychiatric Emergency Room." *Hospital and Community Psychiatry*, 1993, *44*, 782–784.

Ellison, J. M., Hughes, D. H., and White, K. A. "An Emergency Psychiatry Update." *Hospital and Community Psychiatry*, 1989, *40*, 250–260.

Galanter, M., Castaneda, R., and Ferman, J. "Substance Abuse Among General Psychiatric Patients: Place of Presentation, Diagnosis, and Treatment." *American Journal of Drug and Alcohol Abuse*, 1988, *14*, 211–235.

Gillig, P, Dumaine, M., and Hillard, J. R. "Whom Do Mobile Crisis Services Serve?" *Hospital and Community Psychiatry*, 1990, *41*, 804–805.

Gillig, P. M., and others. "What Do Police Officers Really Want from the Mental Health System?" *Hospital and Community Psychiatry*, 1990, *41*, 663–665.

Lamb, H. R. "Public Psychiatry and Prevention." In R. E. Hales, S. C. Yudofsky, and J. A. Talbott (eds.), *The American Psychiatric Press Textbook of Psychiatry.* (2nd ed.) Washington, D.C.: American Psychiatric Press, 1994.

Lamb, H. R. (ed.). *The Homeless Mentally Ill.* Washington, D.C.: American Psychiatric Association, 1984.

Lamb, H. R., and Grant, R. W. "The Mentally Ill in an Urban County Jail." *Archives of General Psychiatry*, 1982, *39*, 17–22.

Lamb, H. R., and Shaner, R. "When There Are Almost No State Hospital Beds Left." *Hospital and Community Psychiatry*, 44, 1993, 973–976.

Lamb, H. R., Sorkin, A. P., and Zusman, J. "Legislating Social Control of the Mentally Ill in California." *American Journal of Psychiatry*, 1981, *138*, 334–339.

Lamb, H. R., and others. "Psychiatric Needs in Local Jails: Emergency Issues." *American Journal of Psychiatry*, 1984, *141*, 774–777.

McNiel, D. E., and Binder, R. L. "Predictive Validity of Judgments of Dangerousness in Emergency Civil Commitment." *American Journal of Psychiatry*, 1987, *144*, 197–200.

McNiel, D. E., and others. "Characteristics of Persons Referred by Police to the Psychiatric Emergency Room." *Hospital and Community Psychiatry*, 1991, *42*, 425–427.

McNiel, D. E., and others. "The Role of Violence in Decisions About Hospitalization from the Psychiatric Emergency Room." *American Journal of Psychiatry*, 1992, *149*, 207–212.

Morrell, L. K. *The Law Enforcement/Mental Health Interface: A Pilot Study of the Impact of Public Policy Changes upon Access to Emergency Psychiatric Services.* Rockville, Md.: National Institute of Mental Health, 1989.

Mulvey, E. P. "Assessing the Evidence of a Link Between Mental Illness and Violence." *Hospital and Community Psychiatry*, 1994, *45*, 663–668.

Sales, G. N. "A Comparison of Referrals by Police and Other Sources to a Psychiatric Emergency Service." *Hospital and Community Psychiatry*, 1991, *42*, 950–952.

Segal, S. P., and others. "Civil Commitment in the Psychiatric Emergency Room: III. Disposition as a Function of Mental Disorder and Dangerousness Indicators." *Archives of General Psychiatry*, 1988, *45*, 759–763.

Szuster, R. R., Schanbacher, B. L., and McCann, S. C. "Characteristics of Psychiatric Emergency Room Patients with Alcohol- or Drug-Induced Disorders." *Hospital and Community Psychiatry*, 1990, *41*, 1342–1345.

Torrey, E. F. "Violent Behavior by Individuals with Serious Mental Illness." *Hospital and Community Psychiatry*, 1994, *45*, 653–662.

Torrey, E. F., and others. "Criminalizing the Seriously Mentally Ill: The Abuse of Jails as Mental Hospitals." *Innovations and Research*, 1993, *2*, 11–14.

Watson, M. A., Segal, S. P., and Newhill, C. E. "Police Referral to Psychiatric Emergency Services and Its Effect on Disposition Decisions." *Hospital and Community Psychiatry*, 1993, *44*, 1085–1090.

Way, B. B., Evans, M. E., and Banks, S. M. "Factors Predicting Referral to Inpatient or Outpatient Treatment from Psychiatric Emergency Services." *Hospital and Community Psychiatry*, 1992, *43*, 703–708.

Way, B. B., Evans, M. E., and Banks, S. M. "An Analysis of Police Referrals to 10 Psychiatric Emergency Rooms." *Bulletin of the American Academy of Psychiatry and the Law, 21*, 1993, 389–397.

Zealberg, J. J., Santos, A. B., and Fisher, R. K. "Benefits of Mobile Crisis Programs." *Hospital and Community Psychiatry*, 1993, *44*, 16–17.

Zealberg, J. J., and others. "A Mobile Crisis Program: Collaboration Between Emergency Psychiatric Services and Police." *Hospital and Community Psychiatry*, 1992, *43*, 612–615.

H. RICHARD LAMB *is professor of psychiatry and the behavioral sciences at Keck School of Medicine, University of Southern California, in Los Angeles.*

RODERICK SHANER *is associate professor of clinical psychiatry at Keck School of Medicine at the University of Southern California, in Los Angeles, and medical director of the Los Angeles County Department of Mental Health.*

DIANA M. ELLIOTT *is clinical associate professor of psychiatry and the behavioral sciences at Keck School of Medicine, University of Southern California, in Los Angeles.*

WALTER J. DECUIR JR. *was detective and officer-in-charge of the mental evaluation unit of the Los Angeles Police Department. He is now retired.*

JAMES T. FOLTZ *is program manager, psychiatric continuing care, with the Los Angeles County Department of Mental Health.*

Mental health consultation is provided to a municipal court that recommends court-mandated interventions for mentally ill persons who have committed minor crimes. This study demonstrates that a significantly better outcome results when the judge not only mandates but monitors mental health treatment.

Court Intervention to Address the Mental Health Needs of Mentally Ill Offenders

H. Richard Lamb, Linda E. Weinberger, Cynthia Reston-Parham

Criminalization of chronically and severely mentally ill persons is a pressing problem (Lamb and Grant, 1982; Hoffman, 1990; Miller, 1992; Torrey and others, 1993; Draine, Solomon, and Meyerson, 1994; Lamb and others, 1995). Criminalization refers to placing mentally ill persons who have committed minor crimes into the criminal justice system instead of into the mental health system, in psychiatric hospitals or other psychiatric treatment facilities.

How did criminalization come about? Before deinstitutionalization, most mentally ill persons who committed minor offenses resided permanently, or for long periods, in state hospitals and thus were not in the community, where their actions could bring them to the attention of the police (Lamb and Grant, 1982; Teplin, 1983). Many writers believe that because of more restrictive commitment standards, mentally ill people are less likely to enter the mental health system; instead, because of their actions and because society has a limited tolerance for them in the community, they are shunted into the criminal justice system (Miller, 1992; Rogers and Bagby, 1992). Other writers believe that a large proportion of the mentally ill who are charged with minor crimes are also among the more difficult to treat; therefore, the mental health system resists treating them, leaving their disposition, and treatment, if any, to the criminal justice system (Draine, Solomon, and Meyerson, 1994).

One approach advocated for stemming the tide of criminalization of mentally ill persons charged with misdemeanors is the provision of mental

Source: Lamb, H. R., Weinberger, L. E., and Reston-Parham, C. "Court Intervention to Address the Mental Health Needs of Mentally Ill Offenders." *Psychiatric Services*, 1996, 47 (3), 275–281. Reprinted by permission.

health consultation to the courts. Consultation, which generally includes the psychiatric evaluation of mentally ill defendants, could be used to divert such persons into the mental health system or at least find suitable psychiatric treatment for them while they remain in the criminal justice system (Joseph and Potter, 1993).

Diversion of the mentally ill person from the criminal justice system to the mental health system can take place at several time points. On the streets, the police can use their discretion to divert to a mental health facility instead of to jail someone they have probable cause to believe has committed a crime. Diversion may also take place at the arraignment court, at the behest of the defense attorney and at the discretion of the judge and prosecuting attorney. Or it may take place later, when the defendant is awaiting trial and residing in jail. However, few diversion programs for mentally ill jail detainees exist at this time (Steadman, Barbera, and Dennis, 1994).

Other forms of diversion, formal diversion or informal diversion, may occur still later, at the time of sentencing or other court disposition.

Formal diversion refers to imposing on a defendant a number of conditions, which may include attending and participating in psychiatric treatment in the mental health system for a specified length of time (Cooke, 1991, 1994). In California, prosecution is postponed so the mentally ill misdemeanant can complete a specified treatment program; if the individual successfully fulfills the conditions imposed by the judge, the criminal charges are dismissed, and "the arrest upon which the diversion was based shall be deemed to never have occurred" (California Penal Code, sec. 1001.9). Some writers have opposed formal diversion, believing it means that the punishment demanded by society is not obtained and that offenders are being treated too leniently (Sanders, 1988; Light, 1986).

Informal diversion occurs as part of the sentencing of a convicted person. It refers to sentencing a mentally disordered offender to mental health treatment as a condition of probation, accompanied by a reduction in or elimination of punishment. The treatment is usually offered through the mental health system rather than the criminal justice system.

It has been observed that because commitment is now more difficult to obtain, involuntary treatment of mentally ill persons today is being obtained in the criminal justice system (Solomon and others, 1995; Awad and Perillo, 1988). Miller (1992) has noted that many civil libertarians feel reassured by the procedural protections of the criminal justice system and are less concerned about the person's acquiring a criminal identity and about other ramifications of entering into a criminal, rather than a civil, mental health system.

Other writers have observed that court-ordered involuntary treatment, such as treatment as a condition of probation, can be effective (Hoffman, 1990; Mendelson, 1992; Brennan and others, 1987). Court-ordered involuntary treatment has been looked on favorably by many persons.

The purpose of this chapter is to examine the outcomes of mental health consultation provided to a municipal court and the court's resulting interventions for mentally ill persons who committed minor crimes. The chapter reports a study of ninety-six mentally ill offenders who were evaluated by a clinical psychologist court consultant and their outcomes one year after arrest. Case examples illustrate the effects of various interventions.

Methods

The Study Site. In 1983, the Los Angeles County Department of Mental Health established a forensic mental health court diversion program to provide mental health expertise and services to the judicial system. One aim of the program is to offer mental health consultation to the courts at an early stage in the defendants' legal process. Another is to divert mentally ill persons from receiving punishment in the criminal justice system to obtaining treatment from the mental health system when appropriate. A defendant is granted formal or informal diversion only after a mental health recommendation for such a disposition.

The Hollywood Municipal Court was chosen as the study site because it had a well-established program of mental health consultation, provided by a clinical psychologist, for the judges, defense attorneys, and city attorneys assigned to the court. Any of these court personnel can refer a defendant for consultation, but the referral is made through the defense attorney. The same psychologist (the third author of this chapter) was the court consultant throughout the study.

Clients who accept the program's services receive an evaluation by the clinical psychologist, which includes a clinical interview and review of the client's mental health and criminal justice records as provided by defense counsel. A treatment plan is developed after collaboration with the client, defense and prosecution attorneys, interested family members, and public and private mental health professionals and is presented to the court. The psychologist also locates appropriate treatment and residential facilities and refers defendants to them. Persons who refuse this service typically do not have mental health consultation offered at their trial.

The clinical psychologist consultant routinely conducts follow-up evaluation of clients, to determine the value of the consultation service. Follow-up consists of review of data added to the client's mental health and criminal justice records after the court disposition, periodic contact with the client, frequent communication with court personnel and professionals from the department of mental health, and, in some cases, contact with the client's family.

Study Subjects and Procedures. The study sample consisted of one hundred persons charged with misdemeanors who were referred to the clinical psychologist for evaluation and who consented to the service. The subjects were chosen at random from the 836 defendants who received court dispositions from August 1990 to October 1993.

For the study, records of the routine evaluation of the subjects were reviewed, as was the subjects' status during the year after the court's disposition. Follow-up information was not available on four subjects during the year; two had left the state, and two had left the country. Thus, the study sample numbered ninety-six subjects.

Subjects were classified as having either a good or a poor outcome during the one-year follow-up. A poor outcome was defined as the occurrence of one or more of the following events during the follow-up year: psychiatric hospitalization, arrest, significant physical violence against persons, and homelessness at the end of the one-year follow-up. Good outcome was defined as the absence of all of those events during the follow-up year.

The study was conducted under the auspices of the Los Angeles County Department of Mental Health, with the approval of the Hollywood division of the Los Angeles County Municipal Court, the Los Angeles County Public Defender's Office, and the Los Angeles City Attorney's Office.

Results

Characteristics of the Subjects at Arrest. The ninety-six subjects ranged in age from 18 to 84 (median, 33.5 years). Sixty-eight (71 percent) were men. Their educational levels ranged from the fifth grade to four years of graduate school (median, four years of high school). Other characteristics of the subjects at the time of evaluation are summarized in Table 6.1.

Subjects tended to be single and to have a history of prior arrest and a history of violence against persons. They tended to have major overt psychopathology (delusions, hallucinations, thought disorder, and similar symptoms) and to have received previous inpatient psychiatric treatment. More than half had a primary diagnosis of a schizophrenic disorder and a history of serious substance abuse.

Table 6.2 lists the charges on which the subjects were arrested preceding the consultation. The most common charge was assault and battery, for forty-one subjects (43 percent). When other crimes of violence against persons are added—three charges of domestic violence and one each of robbery and molesting children—a total of forty-six subjects (48 percent) were arrested on charges of crimes of violence against persons.

Treatment Related to Disposition. For the ninety-six subjects, the mean length of time between arrest and court disposition (that is, sentencing or dismissal) was 2.7 months. Of the eighty persons who spent time in jail during that period, the mean length was 19.8 days.

Fifty-one of the subjects (53 percent) received mental health treatment after their arrest and before their court disposition. Of these fifty-one subjects, fifteen (29 percent) received no treatment after court disposition; some of the fifteen cases were dismissed, some of the subjects had been hospitalized long enough that the court believed they had served a period appropriate for their crime, and for some the judge saw no need to stipulate

Table 6.1. Characteristics of Ninety-Six Defendants in a Municipal Court Who Were Evaluated by a Forensic Mental Health Program

Characteristic	Number	Percentage
Race		
Caucasian	43	45
African American	30	31
Hispanic	13	14
Asian	8	8
Native American	2	2
Marital status		
Single	74	77
Divorced or separated	16	17
Married	5	5
Widowed	1	1
Primary *DSM-III-R* diagnosis		
Schizophrenic disorder	55	57
Bipolar disorder	12	13
Major depression	10	10
Psychotic disorder not otherwise specified	6	6
Organic mental disorder	6	6
Schizoaffective disorder	1	1
Other	6	6
Source of financial support		
Supplemental Security Income	47	49
Employment	17	18
General relief	7	7
Family	4	4
Social Security Disability Insurance	3	3
Other	6	6
No known support	12	13
Prior arrest	68	71
Crimes against persons	39	41
Other crimes	29	30
Treatment history		
Psychiatric hospitalization	66	69
Outpatient treatment	61	64
Conservatorship for grave disability	8	8
Residence in a board-and-care home	16	17
Living situation at arrest		
Homeless	27	28
Alone	18	19
With spouse	17	18
With family	12	13
Board-and-care home	8	8
Rented room, hotel	7	7
With roommate	5	5
Other	2	2
History of physical violence against persons	70	73
History of serious substance abuse	51	53
Major overt psychopathology	81	84

Table 6.2. Charges on Arrest of Ninety-Six Defendants Evaluated by a Forensic Mental Health Program

Charge	Number	Percentage
Assault, battery	41	43
Shoplifting, petty theft	10	10
Trespassing	9	9
Vandalism	8	8
Domestic violence	3	3
Brandishing a weapon	3	3
Burglary	3	3
Exposing self, lewd conduct	3	3
False emergency report	3	3
Violating a restraining order	3	3
Terrorist threats	2	2
Prostitution	2	2
Robbery	1	1
Molesting children	1	1
Child endangerment	1	1
Stalking	1	1
Other	2	2

treatment in the disposition. In all fifteen cases, the treatment before court disposition consisted of psychiatric hospitalization for treatment of psychosis.

At court disposition, fifty-six of the ninety-six subjects (58 percent) were mandated to receive judicially monitored mental health treatment. Eight of these subjects were placed on formal diversion by the judge. Of the other forty-eight subjects mandated to receive judicially monitored treatment, thirty-eight subjects (including four placed in psychiatric hospitals) were to be monitored by the municipal court itself after sentencing; eight were placed on psychiatric conservatorship because of grave disability, and their treatment was monitored by their conservators; and two who were already on parole at the time of the arrest were referred back to their parole officers, who reinstated them in treatment at the parole psychiatric outpatient clinic.

The remaining forty subjects (42 percent) were not mandated to receive monitored treatment after sentencing. For twelve subjects (13 percent), the judge simply dismissed the case. Thirteen subjects (14 percent) received a jail sentence or jail and probation. Fifteen subjects (16 percent) were referred to mental health treatment but without any follow-up monitoring by the court. Of these fifteen, three refused treatment, five became involved in and remained in treatment, and seven dropped out of treatment.

No significant differences were found between the fifty-six subjects mandated to receive monitored treatment and the forty not mandated to receive monitored treatment in terms of age, race, sex, diagnosis, prior arrest history, prior arrests for crimes against persons, prior hospitalizations, living situation, history of physical violence, substance abuse, and presence of major psychopathology. On the same variables, no significant differences were found between the fifty-six subjects mandated to receive monitored treatment and the fifteen who were referred to treatment but not monitored.

Besides mandating treatment or referring subjects for treatment, the court imposed other conditions on many of the defendants who were sentenced. The conditions included jail time for fifty-one subjects (median time, forty days), summary probation for fifty-nine defendants (range, twelve to thirty-six months), a restraining order for sixteen defendants, and community service or payment of restitution for nine defendants.

Outcomes at Follow-Up. As noted, subjects were considered to have a poor outcome if during the year after arrest they had been psychiatrically hospitalized or arrested, had committed significant physical violence against persons, or were homeless at the end of the year. Good outcome was the absence of any of those events. By those criteria, forty-four subjects (46 percent) had a good outcome, and fifty-two (54 percent) had a poor outcome.

A significantly larger proportion of subjects who were mandated to receive judicially monitored treatment had a good outcome compared with subjects who were not mandated to receive monitored treatment ($\chi^2 = 9.28$, df = 1, $p < .01$). Of the fifty-six subjects mandated to receive monitored treatment, thirty-three subjects (59 percent) had a good outcome, and twenty-three (41 percent) had a poor outcome. Of the forty subjects not mandated to receive monitored treatment, eleven (28 percent) had a good outcome, and twenty-nine (72 percent) had a poor outcome.

In addition, subjects mandated to receive judicially monitored treatment had significantly better outcomes than subjects who were referred for treatment but without court monitoring ($\chi^2 = 5.78$, corrected for continuity; df = 1, $p < .02$). Of the latter group of fifteen subjects, three (20 percent) had a good outcome, and twelve (80 percent) had a poor outcome.

When the four criteria for poor outcome are considered individually, the results show that during the one-year follow-up, thirty-three of the ninety-six subjects (34 percent) were psychiatrically hospitalized. The median length of time from court disposition to hospitalization was 3.5 months. Thirty-seven subjects (39 percent) were rearrested. The median length of time from court disposition to arrest was 5.0 months. Sixteen subjects (17 percent) demonstrated significant physical violence against others. At the conclusion of the one-year follow-up period, eleven of the ninety-six subjects (11 percent) were homeless.

Discussion

The Program Overall. This study was a one-year follow-up of ninety-six mentally ill defendants who were arrested for misdemeanors and were referred for and accepted psychiatric evaluation by a clinical psychologist court consultant. Using a single mental health evaluator of course has some limitations. Nevertheless, this study revealed a sample that clearly presented a challenge in management and treatment: the great majority had major overt psychopathology and a diagnosis of schizophrenia or major mood disorder at the time of the arrest; the typical client had prior arrests, a history of physical violence against persons, and prior psychiatric hospitalizations; the charge against almost half of the subjects was some form of violence against persons; and more than one-fourth were homeless at the time of arrest.

Almost three-fifths of the defendants received formal or informal diversion from the criminal justice system and were mandated by the court to receive judicially monitored mental health treatment. A significant relationship was found between monitored mental health treatment and good outcome during the year after sentencing. It should be noted, however, that the subjects were not randomly assigned to monitored treatment versus other dispositions. Rather, the court dispositions were based on judicial decision making.

Overall, the study suggests that several factors are involved in achieving good outcomes for many mentally ill persons who commit minor crimes. First of all, it is important for nonclinicians in the criminal justice system to have assistance in recognizing and diagnosing mental illness and then in making appropriate dispositions. Thus, the court should have readily available consultation from mental health professionals when considering diversion. Furthermore, if the judge is considering mental health treatment as a condition for reducing or eliminating punishment, then, to the extent justified by the law and the nature of the offense, the judge should mandate, not just recommend, that the defendant attend treatment. The judge should also monitor the treatment on an ongoing basis.

One might extrapolate that in many cases, the judge should also mandate an appropriate living situation. If indicated, the living situation might have varying degrees of structure, such as that provided in a supervised apartment program, a residential rehabilitation facility, a group or board-and-care home, or even a locked facility. In any case, the consultation provided by the mental health professional is essential if judges are to understand the psychological condition and needs of the client and to find appropriate treatment programs and living situations.

Once the court makes a mental health referral, the treatment program should accept the responsibility to provide treatment and should apprise the judge of the client's progress and compliance. The mental health program should also, when indicated, make arrangements for an appropriate living situation (supervised if need be) during treatment and at the client's discharge and should apprise the judge of living arrangements too.

Moreover, in keeping with good case management, the treatment team should evaluate and make any necessary arrangements for other aspects of the client's support system during treatment and at discharge, such as ensuring adequate finances and involving the client's family and friends in ongoing care.

Outpatient treatment, including prescription of oral medications, is insufficient for many mentally ill offenders. They may need day treatment or residential treatment, perhaps in a locked twenty-four-hour facility; intramuscular antipsychotic medication; designation of others to control their monies; and, in some cases, psychiatric conservatorship based on grave disability.

It should be recognized that some mentally ill defendants are not appropriate candidates for formal diversion or for court-ordered treatment after sentencing (informal diversion) because of the nature and seriousness of their crime, their inability to profit from treatment, and the lack of resources to treat and monitor them properly. In addition, some defendants may not be willing to accept treatment-related court dispositions. Civil libertarians maintain that mentally ill offenders are within their rights to refuse to cooperate with court-imposed treatment even if refusal may result in jail or some other punitive measure. In fact, some mentally ill defendants choose this course over accepting their mental illness and need for treatment. In some cases, this choice contributes to their criminalization.

Case Examples. Four case examples illustrate the role of a court consultation program and some of the difficulties encountered in the evaluation, disposition, and treatment of mentally ill offenders. Identifying information and some data have been altered to maintain the subjects' anonymity.

Case 1. Mr. B, a thirty-two-year-old single man, was arrested for taking $150 from someone coming out of a bank. Mr. B, who had previously been arrested for the same crime, had experienced multiple psychiatric hospitalizations. He had been diagnosed for the past ten years as having schizophrenic disorder, chronic paranoid type, and cocaine addiction. He was living on the streets.

Mr. B pleaded nolo contendere. He was given twenty-four months' summary probation and was ordered, on the recommendation of the clinical psychologist court consultant, to spend six months at a locked psychiatric facility and then to receive neuroleptic medications on an outpatient basis. At the end of his treatment at the residential facility, the staff there arranged for him to live with his brother and attend outpatient treatment at a local mental health clinic.

The court continued to follow Mr. B's progress regularly while he was living in the community. At the clinic, because of previous poor compliance with medications, Mr. B was given intramuscular fluphenazine. He was randomly tested for illicit drug use and was referred to Narcotics Anonymous. Mr. B's brother was highly supportive of his treatment, and the treatment staff met with both Mr. B and his brother frequently.

At the end of the one-year follow-up period, Mr. B was doing well. Although he was not working, he had not been arrested or hospitalized, he was living with his brother, and he was continuing his treatment.

This case of a monitored informal diversion plan reflects a successful outcome highlighting the impact of several factors. The court recognized the importance of mental health consultation and followed the recommendations of the clinical psychologist consultant. It also remained involved in monitoring the defendant's treatment progress and living situation after sentencing. Furthermore, the inpatient and outpatient treatment programs accepted the responsibility of providing treatment and good case management, which included drug monitoring and arranging for Mr. B's living situation. Having a supportive family member who was active in the treatment was another positive factor.

Case 2. Ms. C was a forty-three-year-old divorced woman who was in the United States on a visitor's visa from a European country and was arrested for trespassing. She had followed a celebrity throughout Europe and the United States, believing she was his wife, and was arrested when she would not leave his home in Los Angeles.

In Europe, Ms. C worked as an engineer and supported herself through monies she invested. She had a history of psychiatric treatment abroad, including multiple hospitalizations, and had been diagnosed as having schizophrenia. She had always refused outpatient psychiatric treatment. Before her arrest in the United States, Ms. C had been arrested two months earlier for a similar offense.

The clinical psychologist consultant referred Ms. C to see the jail psychiatrist, but the defendant refused the referral. Ms. C pleaded nolo contendere, and the judge sentenced her to thirty-six months' summary probation and forty-five days in jail minus time already served. The judge also issued a restraining order for her to stay away from the celebrity.

Ms. C returned to her rented room in Los Angeles, where she lived alone. She had no family or friends in this country. Within a month and a half, she disobeyed the restraining order, was arrested, and was remanded to custody. For this new offense, she was sentenced to 180 days in jail. She served approximately a third of her sentence and was released on probation, with the restraining order reinstated.

Soon afterward, Ms. C followed the celebrity to another state, where she was rearrested and eventually deported. During the one-year follow-up period, she had no psychiatric hospitalizations, nor did she participate in psychiatric outpatient treatment.

In this case, the judge did not attempt to institute any form of diversion with mental health treatment. Given Ms. C's severe psychiatric disturbance, her history of refusing treatment, her lack of any support system, her highly recidivistic behavior, and the threat the victim may have perceived from her actions, the court should have imposed judicially monitored treatment in a residential psychiatric facility. Ms. C could have refused such court-mandated treatment and instead have gone to jail. Even so, the court recognized the high likelihood that Ms. C would commit another offense; therefore, simply placing her under a restraining order and on probation were insufficient deterrents for her.

Case 3. Mr. G was a thirty-seven-year-old single man with a long history of psychiatric hospitalizations and a diagnosis of bipolar disorder. He also manifested severe cocaine and alcohol abuse. He was arrested for stealing food worth twenty-five dollars from a store. At the time of his arrest, Mr. G was attending outpatient treatment, but was generally noncompliant in taking his medications. He was estranged from his family and was living with a woman he had met six months earlier. Over the past six years, he had been arrested on a variety of charges, including battery, exhibiting a deadly weapon, and possession of narcotics.

In court, the judge offered Mr. G a formal diversion plan for six months, which he accepted. On the advice of the clinical psychologist court consultant, the judge ordered him to continue attending the mental health clinic and to comply with the clinic's treatment recommendations, including medications. The judge also ordered him to provide eighty hours of community service, appear before the court with proof that he had completed the community service, and return periodically with progress reports about his mental health treatment.

Mr. G completed his community service obligation, attended and cooperated with the treatment, and produced periodic progress reports for the judge. Six months after Mr. G was placed on diversion, the court ruled that he had successfully completed the conditions of his diversion, and the charges were dismissed. Following the dismissal, Mr. G stopped attending treatment and was soon rearrested on a charge of battery. He was hospitalized for depression several times during the remainder of the one-year follow-up.

This client did well as long as he was in a diversion program under the jurisdiction of the court. However, the minor nature of the offense for which he was arrested, stealing food, limited the length of time that the court could exert social control. After Mr. G's case was dismissed, the mental health clinic should have accepted the responsibility of continuing to provide outreach case management for this chronically and severely mentally ill and potentially dangerous client and to involve his girlfriend in his treatment.

Case 4. Mr. M was a forty-year-old divorced male who was homeless and living in a park at the time of his arrest. He was apprehended by a security officer for stealing flashlight batteries from a grocery store. Mr. M had a history of previous arrests for similar offenses and was on probation at the time of the current arrest. He stated that when he was hungry and tired of living on the streets, he committed petty thefts in order to get arrested.

Mr. M had no documented history of psychiatric treatment but had a long history of polysubstance abuse. He was evaluated by the clinical psychologist court consultant, who made a diagnosis of bipolar disorder and recommended outpatient treatment.

Mr. M pleaded nolo contendere. The court recommended, but did not mandate, psychiatric outpatient treatment. The defendant predictably refused to accept the treatment recommendation, and the judge then sentenced him to ninety days in jail. Mr. M served two months in jail, and on his release the psychologist court consultant provided him with a referral for outpatient treatment. However, Mr. M again denied that he was ill and refused the referral.

The client went to live with an uncle, who found him a part-time job and tried to arrange a suitable living situation. However, Mr. M left his uncle's home and returned to living on the streets. He supported himself through general relief funds and odd jobs, but spent much of the money on drugs. Within four months of his release from jail, Mr. M stole a small radio. At the end of the one-year follow-up period, he was homeless.

This case is an instance of the criminalization of the mentally ill. Left to his own devices, Mr. M appeared to choose the criminal justice system to meet his needs when he could not meet them himself. Moreover, he refused recommendations and help from family and others when it involved the mental health system because he denied that he was mentally ill. Thus, the court felt obliged to take some action, in this case jail.

Would a mandated therapeutic living situation and psychiatric treatment, with the requirement for periodic reports to the court, have made a difference for Mr. M? One cannot say, but it might well have been more beneficial to have attempted such a mental health intervention, with limits and structure imposed by the court, rather than simply placing Mr. M in jail. However, the defendant probably still would have refused these court-mandated interventions, leaving the judge little alternative but to impose criminal sanctions.

Conclusion

This study has shown that court-mandated and court-monitored mental health treatment can be effective in obtaining a good outcome for chronically and severely mentally ill persons who have committed minor crimes, an outcome defined as avoiding rehospitalization, rearrests, physical violence against persons, and homelessness. Using mental health consultation as soon as mentally ill defendants enter the criminal justice system gives the court an opportunity to make a significant impact on this population.

We believe the court should act in the best interests of such mentally ill persons by exerting its powers to mandate mental health treatment, both inpatient and outpatient, and to monitor the individual's progress. We recognize that the civil justice system no longer can exert this leverage with many mentally ill people and that they are receiving judicially what in many cases may amount to involuntary mental health treatment. Is this a legitimate function of the criminal justice system? We believe it is, for, as we see it, it is the court's obligation not simply to punish but to take action to reduce mentally ill individuals' potential to commit other offenses.

References

Awad, G. A., and Perillo, C. "The Court as a Catalyst in the Treatment Process." *American Journal of Psychotherapy*, 1988, 42, 290–296.

Brennan, T. P., and others. "A Vision for Probation and Court Services: Forensic Social Work: Practice and Vision." *Federal Probation*, 1987, 51, 63–70.

California. California Penal Code, sec. 1001.9.

Cooke, D. J. "Treatment as an Alternative to Prosecution: Offenders Diverted for Treatment." *British Journal of Psychiatry*, 1991, *158*, 785–791.

Cooke, D. J. "Primary Diversion for Psychological Treatment: The Decision Making of Procurators Fiscal." *International Journal of Law and Psychiatry*, 1994, *17*, 211–223.

Draine, J., Solomon, P., and Meyerson, A. "Predictors of Reincarceration Among Patients Who Received Psychiatric Services in Jail." *Hospital and Community Psychiatry*, 1994, *45*, 163–167.

Hoffman, B. F. "The Criminalization of the Mentally Ill." *Canadian Journal of Psychiatry*, 1990, *35*, 166–169.

Joseph, P.L.A., and Potter, M. "Diversion from Custody. I: Psychiatric Assessment at the Magistrates' Court." *British Journal of Psychiatry*, 1993, *162*, 325–330.

Lamb, R. H., and Grant, R. W. "The Mentally Ill in an Urban County Jail." *Archives of General Psychiatry*, 1982, *39*, 17–22.

Lamb, H. R., and others. "Outcome for Psychiatric Emergency Patients Seen by a Police–Mental Health Professional Psychiatric Emergency Team." *Psychiatric Services*, 1995, *46*, 1267–1271.

Light, R. "Getting Away with It? Diversion as an Alternative to Prosecution." *New Law Journal*, 1986, *136*, 62–70.

Mendelson, E. F. "A Survey of Practice at a Regional Forensic Service: What Do Forensic Psychiatrists Do? Part II: Treatment, Court Reports, and Outcome." *British Journal of Psychiatry*, 1992, *160*, 773–776.

Miller, R. D. "Economic Factors Leading to Diversion of the Mentally Disordered from the Civil to the Criminal Commitment Systems." *International Journal of Law and Psychiatry*, 1992, *15*, 1–12.

Rogers, R., and Bagby, R. M. "Diversion of Mentally Disordered Offenders: A Legitimate Role for Clinicians?" *Behavioral Sciences and the Law*, 1992, *10*, 407–418.

Sanders, A. "The Limits to Diversion from Prosecution." *British Journal of Criminology*, 1988, *28*, 513–532.

Solomon, P., and others. "Interaction of the Criminal Justice System and Psychiatric Professionals in Which Civil Commitment Standards Are Prohibitive." *Bulletin of the American Academy of Psychiatry and the Law*, 1995, *23*, 117–128.

Steadman, H. J., Barbera, S. S., and Dennis, D. L. "A National Survey of Jail Diversion Programs for Mentally Ill Detainees." *Hospital and Community Psychiatry*, 1994, *45*, 1109–1113.

Teplin, L. "The Criminalization of the Mentally Ill: Speculation in Search of Data." *Psychological Bulletin*, 1983, *94*, 54–67.

Torrey, E. F., and others. "Criminalizing the Seriously Mentally Ill: The Abuse of Jails as Mental Hospitals." *Innovations and Research*, 1993, *2*, 11–14.

H. RICHARD LAMB is professor of psychiatry and the behavioral sciences at Keck School of Medicine, University of Southern California, in Los Angeles.

LINDA E. WEINBERGER is professor of clinical psychiatry and chief psychologist at the Institute of Psychiatry, Law, and Behavioral Sciences at Keck School of Medicine, University of Southern California, in Los Angeles.

CYNTHIA RESTON-PARHAM is clinical psychologist court consultant for the Los Angeles County Department of Mental Health.

7

Mental health conservatorship can play an important role in the clinical management and treatment of persons with severe mental illness.

Therapeutic Use of Conservatorship in the Treatment of Gravely Disabled Psychiatric Patients

H. Richard Lamb, Linda E. Weinberger

The advent of deinstitutionalization has led to a need to conceptualize and develop a comprehensive system for the treatment and management of chronically and severely mentally ill persons in the community. One mechanism, conservatorship, has been shown to be a useful part of an overall strategy of care for some patients in this population.

In our view, conservatorship in California has enabled a number of persons who would otherwise be long-term residents of psychiatric hospitals to live in the community and achieve a considerable measure of autonomy in their lives (Hargreaves and others, 1984; Lamb and Mills, 1986; Young, Mills, and Sack, 1987). On the other hand, conservatorship also provides a means by which those who need intensive twenty-four-hour intermediate or long-term treatment can be hospitalized (Friedman and Savage, 1988; Lamb and Weinberger, 1992).

Little has been published about how conservatorship can be used clinically in the treatment and management of gravely disabled psychiatric patients. The purpose of this chapter is to provide such a clinical perspective.

The Process in California

The provisions for conservatorship of mentally ill persons in California's 1968 Lanterman-Petris-Short Act were intended to "allow another individual or agency to act on the person's behalf and to protect his interests when

Source: Lamb, H. R., and Weinberger, L. E. "Theraputic Use of Conservatorship in the Treatment of Gravely Disabled Psychiatric Patients." *Hospital and Community Psychiatry*, 1993, *44* (2), 147–150. Reprinted by permission.

he is unable to care for himself. The conservator may determine what arrangements are necessary to provide the conservatee with food, clothing, shelter, and further treatment, and he may take any appropriate steps necessary to safeguard the person's property" (California Mental Health Services Act, 1974, p. 23).

In California, conservatorship proceedings are sought for individuals considered "gravely disabled" (California Welfare and Institutions Code, sec. 5000–5466). *Gravely disabled* means "a condition in which a person, as a result of a mental disorder . . . is unable to provide for his or her basic personal needs for food, clothing, or shelter." Conservatorships are granted for a period of one year and can be renewed. The conservatorship can also be terminated before its expiration. The court appoints as a conservator either a private individual or a public agency, such as the public guardian's office.

The conservator may be granted a number of powers over the mentally ill person. Most commonly granted are powers related to the conservatee's residential placement, his or her involvement in psychiatric treatment, and management of the conservatee's money. That is, the conservator has the power to place the conservatee in any setting—for example, at home or in a board-and-care facility, a locked skilled nursing facility, or a psychiatric hospital—and to require that the conservatee participate in psychiatric treatment and take medications in order to remedy or prevent "the recurrence of the conservatee's being gravely disabled" (California Welfare and Institutions Code, sec. 5358).

In previous work, we described persons for whom conservatorship was sought (Lamb and Weinberger, 1992). We assessed the course of sixty subjects over four years in terms of stability (number and length of psychiatric hospitalizations, arrests, serious physical violence, and homelessness) and presence or absence of family support. Family support was defined as family members' close involvement in the patient's treatment, living situations, and financial matters. The subjects' stability appeared to be related to both family support and conservatorship. When one or both were present, patients were significantly more likely to attain stability. For a considerable number of chronically and severely mentally ill persons, conservatorship appeared to play an important role in their clinical management and treatment; it helped to eliminate chaotic lifestyles, movement in and out of hospitals and jails, and life on the streets, particularly when family support was absent.

Generally, patients placed under conservatorship lack internal controls. They need external controls and structure to help them cope with the demands of living in the community without repeated decompensations and exacerbations of illness. These external controls are provided by the powers that the court delegates to the conservator; the powers represent both physical and psychological leverage that can be exerted on the conservatee. This legally sanctioned control helps hold self-destructive tendencies in check and frees the conservatees' energies to respond to treatment and rehabilitation efforts.

Thus far we have discussed the fundamental reasons and theoretical basis for conservatorship. Next we discuss and illustrate three important elements of the therapeutic use of conservatorship: families' use of conservatorship to help stabilize the patient, the need for simultaneous case management for most conservatees, and the use of conservatorship to facilitate necessary inpatient treatment. Four case examples illustrate these concepts and also some of the difficulties in using conservatorship for gravely disabled patients. Minor changes have been made in some of the facts of the cases to preserve confidentiality.

Conservatorship and Family Involvement

Conservatorship may not only play an essential part in the patient's treatment but also may enable the patient's family to become more effective in helping to stabilize the patient. It can also improve the relationship between patient and family by reducing the chaos caused by the illness and alleviating some of the stress on the family. These outcomes are especially likely when clinicians are skilled in using the leverage of conservatorship in their treatment of patients and in instructing families in ways to apply this leverage. The following case highlights these issues.

Case 1. A thirty-seven-year-old man had been hospitalized briefly every year since age twenty-four. His diagnosis was consistently schizophrenia, paranoid type, according to the criteria of the *DSM-III-R*. He had frequently made threats of violence but was not actually violent. The psychiatric hospitalization that resulted in conservatorship was precipitated when the patient attempted to strangle his niece; broke down doors, walls, and windows; and destroyed furniture. He threatened to cut off the heads of family members, and this time the family took his threats very seriously.

When the patient was admitted to the county hospital, the family reluctantly refused to take him back, and a conservatorship was obtained for the first time. The patient's mother was named as conservator. He was transferred, on conservatorship, from the county hospital to the state hospital. The clinical staff worked closely with the family on their feelings of guilt about setting limits on the patient.

After the patient had been treated for eight months in the state hospital, a family conference was held. The family agreed to let him return to living in an apartment behind their home, but only if there was no further violence and he would agree to take his medications. They also emphasized in no uncertain terms that another episode of violence would permanently terminate this arrangement. The patient agreed and returned to the family. He remained a conservatee for another fourteen months, during which time he attended an outpatient clinic and took his medications.

When the patient's conservatorship was up for renewal for a third year, another family conference was held. The family agreed that further conservatorship was not necessary, but made it clear that if the patient stopped his medications or became physically violent, conservatorship would again be sought and the patient could no longer live with the family. Three years after discharge from the hospital, the patient was not on conservatorship, was living in the apartment behind the family home, was eating his meals with the family, and was taking his medications. He had manifested no further decompensations or episodes of physical violence and had experienced the longest period of stability since the onset of the illness.

In this case, the family rejected the patient after he became violent during an acute, severe decompensation. In our clinical experience, it is frequently at the point of physical violence that the family finally ejects a mentally ill relative, often permanently. Here, conservatorship and a lengthy hospitalization in a state hospital setting gave the family a period of respite while the patient was being stabilized. Conservatorship also gave the family a way to exert leverage on the patient to ensure his compliance with treatment, and it reassured them that if they took him back and the violence recurred, there was a mechanism by which he could be promptly removed from their home.

Working with the clinical staff appeared to enable the family to set limits without their previous ambivalence. Moreover, the patient seemed to respond to the limits set; he knew that lack of compliance with his agreement to continue treatment would lead to rehospitalization and probably a reinstitution of conservatorship. The very real possibility that the family might permanently eject him was another important factor. Thus, a combination of conservatorship and family support appeared to be instrumental in stabilizing this patient.

In other situations, an ambivalent family and a clinical staff's lack of skill in using the powers of conservatorship can mean that neither the patient nor the family receives the help they need.

Case 2. A twenty-five-year-old single woman had first been hospitalized at age twenty-two and had undergone multiple hospitalizations in the subsequent three years. Her diagnosis was bipolar disorder, manic (*DSM-III-R*). She also had a serious problem with alcohol and cocaine abuse. In the past, she had struck her grandmother and had been arrested for being drunk in public. The family believed they could no longer manage her at home and arranged for her placement in a board-and-care home.

The patient was hospitalized six months later when she was found wandering near the county hospital shouting, "Praise the Lord," and obstructing traffic. She was acutely manic and uncontrollable. In the hospital, she was placed on neuroleptic medication, and lithium was begun. Some improvement was noted, but her manic behavior continued. In a meeting with the staff in which the options for future treatment and management were discussed, the family expressed a desire to seek a conservatorship. The conservatorship papers were filed. However, on the day of the patient's conservatorship court hearing, the family phoned saying they had changed their minds and wanted the patient to return home. The conservatorship proceeds were dropped, and the patient returned to the family.

After a month, the family again found themselves unable to manage the patient, and she was again placed in a board-and-care home. During the next four years, her course included occasional periods of living on the streets, numerous hospitalizations for manic episodes, and two arrests for petty theft and disturbing the peace, for which she spent brief periods in jail. The patient consistently refused to continue her lithium or any other medications. Although her behavior was manic, she experienced recurrent episodes of acute dysphoria. She also returned to alcohol and cocaine abuse. She was repeatedly sent to live in board-and-care homes, but she could not be managed there and would not remain.

The family continued their involvement with the patient but stated that her behavior was more than they could handle. In spite of all these problems, the family was too ambivalent and felt too guilty to place her under conservatorship.

The patient's life was chaotic from the onset of her illness. The family tried to offer assistance but was usually overwhelmed. We believe a conservatorship should have been obtained because the patient repeatedly demonstrated that she could not cope on her own or be managed by her family. Perhaps a more concerted effort by the hospital staff might have resolved the family's ambivalence about conservatorship, allowing a family member or, if need be, the public guardian to be named conservator. Whether the authority of the court and a conservator's monitoring of her medication, living situation, and money management would have stabilized this patient or whether she would also have needed prolonged twenty-four-hour structured care cannot be determined.

Integrating Conservatorship and Case Management

The integration of modern concepts of clinical case management (Harris and Bachrach, 1988; Lamb, Weinberger, and Gross, 1988) with conservatorship is another important component if community treatment for chronically and severely mentally ill persons who require conservatorship is to succeed. Almost all conservatees need the basic elements of case management, which starts with the premise that each patient has a designated professional with overall responsibility for his or her care.

The case manager formulates an individualized treatment and rehabilitation plan with the participation of both the conservatee and the conservator. The leverage and authority of the court that the conservatorship provides may make it possible to carry out a plan that otherwise could not be implemented. As care progresses, the case manager monitors the conservatee to determine if he or she is receiving treatment, has an appropriate living situation, has adequate funds, and has access to vocational rehabilitation. The case manager provides outreach services and also makes sure the conservatee is not drifting away from the supportive elements of such a network. In exercising their responsibilities, conservators should seek out case management to ensure that conservatees receive proper care and treatment in the community.

Case 3. A thirty-five-year-old divorced man with a history of numerous psychiatric hospitalizations had a *DSM-III-R* diagnosis of schizoaffective disorder. His history included an arrest in another state for assault with a deadly weapon. He also had a long history of hitting other patients in the board-and-care homes where he lived. Poor compliance with medications had been a consistent problem, as was alcohol and drug abuse. On his last hospitalization, he was brought to the hospital by the police after he threatened fellow patients and staff in his board-and-care home with physical violence and exposed himself.

In the hospital, he remained delusional and hyperactive. All of his family lived out of state; they expressed concern but no inclination to become reinvolved with him. A conservatorship was granted, and the public guardian's office was named the conservator. The patient was transferred from the county hospital to the state hospital and remained there until the expiration of the one-year conservatorship period.

At this point, the patient agreed to live in a board-and-care home and take his medications. His conservatorship was not renewed despite his history of doing poorly in such homes. After a few months in the home, he stopped taking his medications and became threatening toward the staff, who asked him to leave. He went to live in missions and occasionally on the streets. He was usually too disorganized to arrange to receive his Supplemental Security Income checks. Three years after termination of his conservatorship, he was living on the streets, chronically delusional and psychotic, still abusing alcohol, and severely depressed.

The outlines of this case are all too common, especially in larger cities. Given the patient's history of poor adjustment in the community and lack of family support, the conservatorship should have been renewed, at least during the transition from hospital to community, to ensure his ongoing stability and compliance with an appropriate treatment plan. Then the patient's conservator should have sought out assertive case management to arrange for the patient's disability benefits, monitor his medications, and see that he was living in a setting with appropriate structure. Unfortunately, this patient was not offered such support and was left to fend for himself in a world with which he could not cope.

Conservatorship and Hospitalization

Conservatorship can be a key factor in helping to maintain chronically and severely mentally ill persons in the community. However, for some patients, community treatment together with conservatorship, no matter how intensive and well conceived, is not enough. Conservatorship can then become a mechanism to facilitate intermediate periods of hospitalization so that the patient achieves stabilization. For other patients, those whose mental illness is so severe that it precludes treatment in a less restrictive setting, conservatorship helps make long-term hospitalization possible.

Case 4. A twenty-seven-year-old single woman had a history of multiple state hospitalizations on the East Coast since age eighteen. Her *DSM-III-R* diagnosis was bipolar disorder. She came to Los Angeles because she had relatives in the area. Besides experiencing acute manic episodes, she abused alcohol and a variety of street drugs. Her relatives soon decided that the patient could not be managed at home and placed her in a board-and-care home.

The patient was brought to the county psychiatric hospital by the police after disrobing and urinating on herself in a church, maintaining that she was Joan of Arc. Her symptoms did not remit, and a conservatorship was obtained, with the public guardian's office named as conservator. After six weeks in the county hospital, the patient was placed in a locked skilled nursing facility that offered special programs for psychiatric patients. This facility was unable to manage her because of her repeated manic episodes, threats toward other patients, and resistance to taking medications. She was transferred to the state hospital, where she remained for twenty-seven months.

Two further attempts at placement ended in decompensation, and it was concluded that this patient required a long-term, highly structured setting for an indefinite period. She was returned to the state hospital, where she continues to live. There are no plans in the foreseeable future to place her in a less structured setting. The patient has now been under conservatorship continuously for more than four years.

This case illustrates the difficulty of managing and treating some severely ill patients in the community, even with continuous conservatorship, thoughtful management, and close supervision. Although attempts were made to place this patient in less restrictive community facilities, she appeared to need a high degree of structure, as is provided in a state hospital, on a continuous basis. Even when the conservatorship process is well executed, it may not be enough to help a very difficult patient maintain community tenure.

Conclusion

If effectively implemented, conservatorship can be a valuable tool in managing and treating a subpopulation of the chronically and severely mentally ill. It is especially important if these gravely disabled persons do not have close family involvement and support. Conservatorship is intended to provide only the external controls and structure that are necessary for successful treatment and management in the community. Furthermore, conservatorship together with case management can be a powerful combination for this group of mentally ill persons. When patients cannot live in the community, even with conservatorship, family support, and good-quality outpatient services, conservatorship facilitates intermediate or long-term hospitalization.

Conservatorship can empower family members, if they are named as conservators, to become an important part of the treatment plan. Conservatorship may give families a way of exerting leverage over the conservatee, with the assistance, one hopes, of skilled clinical staff. The family's leverage may be both physical and psychological and is directed toward treating or preventing the recurrence of the mental illness that led to the patient's grave disability.

Although conservatees have given up some of their independence because of the conservators' power over them, many who would otherwise lose all of their liberty, through long-term hospitalization, are able to retain most of their autonomy and live in the community. Moreover, conservatorship can transform a dangerous, dysphoric, and deprived existence into one that is relatively free of chaos and may well enable the conservatee to derive increased gratification from life.

References

California Mental Health Services Act. Sacramento: California Health and Welfare Agency, 1974.

California Welfare and Institutions Code, secs. 5000–5466.

California Welfare and Institutions Code, sec. 5358.

Friedman, L., and Savage, M. "Taking Care: The Law of Conservatorship in California." Southern California Law Review, 1988, 61, 273–290.

Hargreaves, W. A., and others. "Restrictiveness of Care Among the Severely Mentally Disabled." Hospital and Community Psychiatry, 1984, 35, 706–709.

Harris, M., and Bachrach, L. L. (eds.). Clinical Case Management. New Directions for Mental Health Services, no. 40. San Francisco: Jossey-Bass, 1988.

Lamb, H. R., and Mills, M. J. "Needed Changes in Law and Procedure for the Chronically Mentally Ill." Hospital and Community Psychiatry, 1986, 37, 475–480.

Lamb, H. R., and Weinberger, L. E. "Conservatorship for Gravely Disabled Psychiatric Patients: A Four-Year Follow-Up Study." American Journal of Psychiatry, 1992, 149, 909–913.

Lamb, H. R., Weinberger, L. E., and Gross, B. H. "Court-Mandated Outpatient Treatment for Insanity Acquittees: Clinical Philosophy and Implementation." Hospital and Community Psychiatry, 1988, 39, 1080–1084.

Young, J. L., Mills, M. J., and Sack, R. L. "Civil Commitment by Conservatorship: The Workings of California's Law." Bulletin of the American Academy of Psychiatry and the Law, 1987, 15, 127–139.

H. RICHARD LAMB is professor of psychiatry and the behavioral sciences at Keck School of Medicine, University of Southern California, in Los Angeles.

LINDA E. WEINBERGER is professor of clinical psychiatry and chief psychologist at the Institute of Psychiatry, Law, and Behavioral Sciences at Keck School of Medicine, University of Southern California, in Los Angeles.

After a brief history, this chapter describes important
modalities and models of psychiatric rehabilitation.

A Century and a Half of Psychiatric Rehabilitation in the United States

H. Richard Lamb

Psychiatric rehabilitation has been an integral part of psychiatric treatment in the United States since the beginnings of moral treatment in the early nineteenth century. The practice of psychiatric rehabilitation encompasses several different, but philosophically related, approaches to the care of people with long-term mental illnesses; the central goal is to enable such individuals to develop their capacities to the fullest extent possible (Bachrach, 1992).

Major elements of psychiatric rehabilitation include focusing on the mentally ill person's strengths, improving vocational and social competencies, working with the environmental facets of the mentally ill person's life, and imparting a sense of mastery and hope (Bachrach, 1992; Lamb, 1982). Confusion has existed about the differences between psychiatric rehabilitation and psychosocial rehabilitation; however, Bachrach (1992) has found that the terms appear to be used interchangeably in the current literature.

This chapter offers a broad discussion of developments in psychiatric rehabilitation in the United States over the past 150 years. The first part sketches historical aspects of the field, the second discusses major conceptual underpinnings, the third describes more recent models and modalities, and the final section discusses some current concerns. The chapter uses the term *psychiatric rehabilitation* except where authors who are cited specifically use *psychosocial rehabilitation*.

Historical Framework

The first half of the nineteenth century was marked by the flowering of moral treatment (Bockoven, 1963; Rothman, 1971; Grob, 1973; Mora and Brand,

Source: Lamb, H. R. "A Century and a Half of Psychiatric Rehabilitation in the United States." *Hospital and Community Psychiatry*, 1994, 45 (10), 1015–1020. Reprinted by permission.

1970), which encompassed the first organized psychiatric rehabilitation effort in the United States. In the small private and state hospitals in which moral treatment was practiced, mentally ill patients were treated with compassion and concern. Treatment included three to four hours a day of a variety of leisure activities, social gatherings, educational and religious lectures, and manual labor. The expectation was that such activity would prevent morbid thoughts and reeducate patients for their expected return to their families and communities. Clinicians were optimistic that mental illness could be cured and that the mentally ill could live in society.

In the midst of the moral treatment era, in 1841, Dorothea Lynde Dix began her remarkable forty-year crusade, devoted principally to the goal of building enough "insane asylums" to accommodate all mentally sick persons then confined in penal and pauper institutions (Deutsch, 1944). The shocking conditions that she found in jails and almshouses led her to investigate such places of confinement personally. She made a great point of contrasting the widely prevalent brutality toward and neglect of the mentally ill in jails and almshouses with the humane, therapeutic atmosphere of the few mental hospitals in operation at the time.

As the nineteenth century progressed, the stresses created by the Industrial Revolution and the congregation of more and more people in the cities, as well as the great influx of immigrants to the United States, caused the state hospitals to become more and more overcrowded. New state hospitals became far larger than the 250-person maximum recommended by the advocates of moral treatment. The therapeutic optimism of moral treatment gave way to a pessimistic view that all mental patients suffered from incurable degenerative nervous system illnesses (Borus, 1987). As a result of this view and the sheer size of these institutions, by the end of the nineteenth century most of the state hospitals had become primarily custodial.

Family Care. An important positive development in psychiatric rehabilitation was the introduction of family care in the United States. The prototype was the program founded in the fifteenth century in Geel, Belgium (Carty and Breault, 1967). In the United States in the nineteenth century, family care meant that a hospital placed some of its patients with families other than their own and maintained and supervised them there (Pollock, 1936). Sometimes the patient's family financed this arrangement, but usually it was supported by the hospital.

Massachusetts was the first state to set up family care, in 1885 (Hamilton, 1944). The family care caseload ran between three hundred and four hundred patients. After several decades, the program was adopted by other states and in Ontario, Canada. Family care gave mentally ill persons an opportunity both to live in the community and to experience participating in the life of a family. As a result, some patients were ultimately able to return to their own families.

Adolf Meyer. In the early part of the twentieth century, Adolf Meyer, generally considered the founder of modern psychiatry in the United States (Mora and Brand, 1970), emphasized the need to understand the role of both the social environment and biological factors in determining psychopathology. Included in his "common-sense psychiatry" was an idea essential to psychiatric rehabilitation: that psychiatrists must work with the healthy part of the personality. Meyer supported Clifford Beers (1908) in establishing the mental hygiene movement, whose goals included rehabilitation and whose tenets anticipated many of the principles of the community mental health movement.

The Modern Era of Psychiatric Rehabilitation. In the 1960s and 1970s, publications by Anthony (1980), Liberman (Liberman and others, 1975; Liberman, DeRisi, and Mueser, 1989; Liberman, McCann, and Wallace, 1976), Brown (Brown, Bone, Dalison, and Wing, 1966) Wing (Wing and Morris, 1981), and Lamb (Lamb and Mackota, 1968; Lamb and others, 1971) began to define the contemporary outlines of the field and to develop philosophies and technologies for working with long-term severely mentally ill patients.

An event that is sometimes taken for granted today but that had tremendous impact on modern psychiatry and rehabilitation was the introduction of antipsychotic medications in the 1950s. Maintenance antipsychotic drug treatment has proved to be of enormous value in reducing the risk of psychotic relapse and rehospitalization (Davis, 1975; Davis and others, 1980; Kane and Marder, 1993; Kane and Lieberman, 1987). Without these medications, community rehabilitation and treatment might not be possible for a large number of long-term severely mentally ill persons.

Conceptual Framework

British psychiatrist John Wing (1977) was a major contributor to the conceptual underpinnings of psychiatric rehabilitation. He observed in a speech that for many long-term mentally ill persons, either too many or too few demands create serious problems. "Many patients who experience an attack of acute schizophrenia remain vulnerable to social stresses of two different kinds. On the one hand, too much social stimulation, experienced by the patient as social intrusiveness, may lead to an acute relapse. On the other hand, too little stimulation will exacerbate any tendency already present toward social withdrawal, slowness, underactivity, and an apparent lack of motivation. Thus, the patient has to walk a tightrope between two different types of danger, and it is easy to become decompensated either way."

An important concept in psychiatric rehabilitation is giving mentally ill persons a sense of mastery—that is, the feeling that they can cope with their internal drives, their symptoms, and the demands of their environment (Lamb, 1982). All treatment and rehabilitation should be designed to help patients improve their ability to deal with and master both internal and external demands to the limits of their potential. With the development of mastery, mentally ill persons achieve not only a better adaptation to their world but also a significant rise in self-esteem and sense of self-worth.

Most rehabilitation professionals have come to believe that to attain this objective, they must work with the well part of the person, with the person's strengths rather than deficiencies. Regardless of the extent of psychopathology in evidence, the person always has an intact portion of personality and capabilities to which treatment and rehabilitation can be directed (Lamb and others, 1971). The goal is to expand the remaining well part rather than to remove or cure pathology. When the healthy part of the personality is expanded, the person is better able to function (Beard, Goertzel, and Pearce, 1958).

Important contributors to the development of psychiatric rehabilitation were made by Olshansky (1968), who challenged some long-held assumptions. First, he demonstrated that no clear relationship exists, as many have supposed, between work capacity and degree of emotional recovery; that is, the ability to obtain a job and then perform it does not require a certain degree of wellness. Some of the sickest and most disturbed people are able to work, some of them marginally and some with a high degree of competence.

Second, he pointed out that, contrary to belief, people do not have to be socialized before they are able to work; they do not have to achieve a high enough level of social skills to get along with other people. Some mentally ill persons can act appropriately within a structured work situation where cues are available to guide them, even though in a social situation they may be immobilized and confused by the lack of structure. Others may achieve a high level of social skills but be unable or unwilling to work.

With the exodus of long-term severely mentally ill persons into the community, attention was turned not simply to their symptoms but to their functional capabilities and limitations. As a result, the importance of psychiatric rehabilitation was increasingly recognized (Munich and Lang, 1993). Also recognized was the great variation among persons with long-term severe mental illness. Many can attain relatively high levels of social and vocational functioning, whereas many others are socially isolated, have exaggerated dependency needs, and often manifest profound social and vocational impairments (Dincin, 1975; Simon, 1965; Bellack and Mueser, 1993; Greenblatt, 1962; Dzhagarov, 1937).

Probably the best summation of the philosophy underlying the practice of psychiatric or psychosocial rehabilitation is by Bachrach (1992). She lists eight fundamental concepts that define the field. First, the central goal is to enable an individual who suffers from long-term mental illness to develop to the fullest extent of his or her capacities. She stresses that rehabilitation must be individualized for each person. Second, environmental factors are important; either the mentally ill person must be helped to adapt to environmental realities, or the environment must be changed to suit the person's needs and capabilities.

Third, the primary concern of psychosocial rehabilitation is to improve patients' competency and to work with the strengths or well part of the person. Fourth, psychosocial rehabilitation is eminently positive in its philosophy, with "the aim of restoring hope to individuals who, because of their psychiatric illnesses, have suffered major setbacks in functional capacity and self-esteem" (p. 1457).

Bachrach's fifth essential concept is optimism about the vocational potential of mentally ill individuals. Sixth, psychosocial rehabilitation is not limited to vocational goals but also encompasses social and recreational aspects of living. Included are such activities as social clubs, resocialization programs, and training in social skills. Seventh, mentally ill persons must be actively involved in their own care and if possible in the design of their rehabilitation programs. Eighth, psychosocial rehabilitation is an ongoing process rather than a one-time effort, and continuity of care is emphasized.

Models and Modalities

Among the treatment modalities and models that are currently in prominent use in psychiatric rehabilitation are the day hospital, social skills training, psychoeducation, and the Fountain House model. They illustrate the sophisticated technology that now characterizes the field.

The Day Hospital. The advent of the day hospital or day treatment center was an important development in psychiatric rehabilitation. This "hospital without beds" (Greenblatt, 1962) originated in 1933 in Moscow, where it served eighty patients as a unit of a psychiatric hospital (Dzhagarov, 1937). Patients lived at home and attended the day hospital from 8 A.M. to 6 P.M. They received the same types of treatment as in the full-time hospital, with emphasis on work therapy.

The first day hospital in the Western Hemisphere was established by Donald Cameron (1947) at the Allan Memorial Institute of Psychiatry in Montreal in 1946. In 1948, Joshua Bierer (1951) established the Marlboro Day Hospital at the Institute of Social Psychiatry in Great Britain. An integral part of Bierer's day hospital was the therapeutic social club.

By the late 1950s and early 1960s, more than one hundred day hospitals were established in the United States (Henisz, 1984). Their numbers and prominence were greatly increased by passage of the Community Mental Health Centers Act in 1963, which mandated partial hospitalization as one of five essential elements of the new centers.

The day treatment center came to serve four types of patients: those in crisis, for whom the day center prevents inpatient hospitalization; those in a hospital who can be discharged early only if they can briefly continue treatment in an all-day community program before entering outpatient treatment; those who do not yet need inpatient hospitalization but are at risk of it without day treatment intervention; and long-term patients in the community who have regressed and need an assessment and the formulation of a rehabilitation program (Lamb, 1976).

Attention to Cognitive Deficits. A growing research literature has documented a variety of impairments in information processing in schizophrenia (Neuchterlein and Dawson, 1984b; Braff and others, 1991). Bellack and Mueser (1993) write, "Almost every aspect of cognitive function has been implicated, including memory, ability to focus and sustain attention, processing speed and capacity, reaction time, problem-solving ability, distractibility and sensorimotor gating, concept formation, and the ability to integrate diverse sensory stimuli. There is a voluminous literature on the neural basis, nature, breadth, and depth of these various dysfunctions, and it is generally assumed that they play a central role in the behavioral dysfunctions characteristic of the disorder" (p. 321).

Research is underway to determine how these cognitive deficits affect the rehabilitation process and how rehabilitation strategies should be altered to address the deficits. Studies have already documented that deficits in verbal memory, early visual processing of information, and vigilance serve rate-limiting functions in determining how much and how well individuals with schizophrenia learn skills relevant to community adaptation (Liberman and Green, 1992).

Social Skills Training. The vulnerability-stress-coping-competence model of major mental disorders is widely used by rehabilitation practitioners as a way of understanding symptoms and social functioning as the end result of a complex interaction among biological, environmental, and behavioral factors and as the theoretical structure for designing rehabilitation strategies (Liberman, 1982, 1992; Neuchterlein and Dawson, 1984a; Anthony and Liberman, 1986). In this model, symptoms and associated disabilities may occur when underlying psychological vulnerability factors are triggered (which is more likely in the absence of optimal antipsychotic medications); when stressful life events exceed the individual's coping skills; when the person's social support network weakens or diminishes; or when coping and problem-solving skills atrophy because of disuse, reinforcement of the sick role, or loss of motivation (Anthony and Liberman, 1986).

Social skills training has gained widespread acceptance as an effective psychosocial rehabilitation strategy for dealing with psychiatric symptoms and disabilities. Social skills training involves the systematic application of behavior learning techniques designed to help individuals gain the knowledge and skills they need to perform in social settings. These skills include holding conversations, establishing and maintaining friendships, dating, managing medications and symptoms, and grooming and self-care (Liberman, 1992). Trainer packages for use in teaching social skills are available; they include specific, goal-oriented instructions to be given by the therapist to the patient and instructions for modeling by the therapist of appropriate use of these skills and for reinforcement and directive feedback to be given to the patient (Liberman and others, 1975; Liberman, McCann, and Wallace, 1976; Cohen, Danley, and Nemec, 1986).

Psychoeducation. An important recent contribution to psychiatric rehabilitation is the psychoeducational approach, used with families who have a schizophrenic relative. Mental health professionals impart specific information to family members, often in a small-group setting, about schizophrenia and about ways of dealing with schizophrenic relatives (Falloon and others, 1985; Anderson, Reiss, and Hogarty, 1986; Golstein, 1981). Techniques vary, but the following elements are used by most practitioners. Families are explicitly told that there are no scientific data to suggest that schizophrenia is caused by childhood upbringing or family interactions. Biochemical and genetic theories are outlined in a manner comprehensible to the families. Visual aids and clearly written handouts are used to augment discussion. Families are also given information to help them understand and support the medication regimen of their schizophrenic relative.

It is usually emphasized that the illness includes a vulnerability to the interpersonal stresses common in everyday life. The approach focuses on helping the family identify and develop strategies to deal with the problems that present the greatest threat to their relative's current and future stability.

The family is also told, implicitly or explicitly, that family members should begin to lead independent and satisfying lives and that being self-sacrificing is counterproductive. Families are encouraged to pay a normal amount of attention to the needs of other family members. Failure to do so is likely to deplete family resources and make long-term support of their schizophrenic relative increasingly difficult.

The schizophrenic person's sensitivity to environmental stimulation is emphasized. Families are told how to create barriers to overstimulation by setting reasonable limits, having realistic goals, and allowing for interpersonal distance; the need for distance relates to survival and does not constitute rejection. For instance, time-outs allow the person with schizophrenia or other family members to retreat to their room or go for a walk when they feel agitated or overstimulated.

The Fountain House Model. One of the cornerstones of the modern psychosocial rehabilitation movement, and a model that has been widely emulated, is the Fountain House model, developed by John Beard and his associates (Beard, Propst, and Malamud, 1982; Beard, 1976).

Fountain House is a club that is considered to belong to those who participate in it. The participants are called members. All members are made to feel that their presence is expected, wanted, and welcomed. The program is set up so that it will not work without the cooperation of its members, and in fact it would collapse without their contributions. In the prevocational day program, members work together with staff in preparing and serving food, keeping the facility clean, doing clerical work, operating the telephones, and publishing a daily newspaper or monthly magazine. Some with special academic skills tutor fellow members, and others work in the thrift shop.

The transitional employment program places members in normal places of business; each member works half-time in an entry-level job, under the supervision of Fountain House staff, to enhance job skills and gain work experience. Fountain House also operates an evening and weekend social-recreational program to improve members' social skills, decrease their isolation, and enable them to maintain long-term contact with the clubhouse after they have become fully employed. This mechanism enables members to continue to benefit from the supportive relationships developed at Fountain House.

An apartment program, which was probably the country's first satellite housing program, provides less institutional, more normalized housing alternatives for members. Fountain House also focuses on helping members maintain themselves on prescribed medication and ensuring that they get required psychiatric care.

Current Issues

As would be expected, a lack of consensus exists about some issues in the field of psychiatric rehabilitation, reflecting conceptual differences among practitioners.

Overselling Rehabilitation. The exodus of the hundreds of thousands of mentally ill persons from the state hospitals into the community that began in the 1950s was at first greeted with enthusiasm. However, by the early 1970s, many recognized that large numbers of long-term severely mentally ill persons were living impoverished lives in the community (Lamb and Goertzel, 1971). One result was an outcry for an array of services—to improve the quality of their lives, raise the level of their social and vocational functioning, integrate them into community life, and give them identities of citizen, worker, or student rather than simply of mental patient.

Paul and Lentz (1977) demonstrated that intensive psychosocial intervention in the form of social learning therapy could significantly improve chronically institutionalized patients' self-care, interpersonal and communication skills, and general level of in-hospital functioning. Social learning therapy also brought a corresponding reduction in bizarre behavior, as well as a greater likelihood of release to the community. Paul and Lentz's purpose was to prepare such patients for at least a partly independent life in the community after discharge from the hospital.

Similarly, mental health professionals increasingly recognized that social and vocational rehabilitation in the community can significantly improve the quality of life for many persons with long-term severe mental illness. Having no reason to get up in the morning and no structured day to look forward to are great voids in their lives; for many, rehabilitation can help fill the voids.

Thus, there was a growing realization that mental health professionals should offer rehabilitation to mentally ill persons, make it attractive for them, and urge them to participate. However, the result in some instances was a shift from virtual neglect to overenthusiastic attempts at rehabilitation and unrealistic expectations. It became clear that if patients cannot cope and if they start to become symptomatic or to run from rehabilitative efforts, professionals need to come to terms with their own therapeutic ambitions, reduce pressure on patients, and learn how to let them decline such activities gracefully and without fear of censure.

Professionals became increasingly aware that they themselves must maintain realistic expectations based on careful assessment of patients' ability to handle various kinds of stress (Lamb and others, 1971). Many professionals began to recognize that they ran the risk of discrediting rehabilitation if they oversold it and made promises they could not keep (Lamb, 1982).

Differences in Rehabilitation Between the United States and the United Kingdom. Shepherd (1991), a British psychiatrist, has noted a difference in emphasis between American and English rehabilitation practitioners. Americans emphasize skills acquisition and the importance of a skills-based approach in helping people function as independently as possible with the minimum of support (Anthony, 1980; Anthony, Cohen, and Cohen, 1984). In contrast, the English focus on understanding the factors that contribute to high-quality, long-term care and helping people adapt despite their disabilities; skills acquisition tends to have an important but secondary role (Shepherd, 1991, 1988; Allen, Gillespie, and Hall, 1989). Shepherd writes:

> What is important in determining a person's social adaptation is the dynamic interaction between his or her disabilities and their social environment. Psychiatric rehabilitation addresses this dynamic adaptation and attempts to maximize functioning, while at the same time acknowledging the possibility of relatively fixed disabilities and the necessity of providing supportive environments.
>
> This dynamic view of the nature of psychological adaptation stands in sharp contrast to the traditional concept of rehabilitation which sees it as a process of "throughput" whereby patients are 'rehabilitated' through attempts to improve their functioning so that they will eventually be able to lead relatively independent lives. The 'adaptive' view of rehabilitation sees attempts to improve functioning as part of the rehabilitation process, but not as synonymous with it. Thus, patients may be successfully 'rehabilitated,' yet remain in a very sheltered, highly dependent setting (i.e. in hospital). Hence, a clear distinction is made between 'rehabilitation' and 'resettlement': successful rehabilitation may include the process of resettlement, but also it may not.
>
> The criterion of successful rehabilitation is that the individual achieves the best adaptation that he or she is capable of and this may, or may not, rest on significant improvements in functioning. In the most extreme cases it may only mean a reduction in the rate of deterioration. This still constitutes successful rehabilitation [pp. xiii-xiv].

To what extent are these differences between countries real or semantic? A debate of the issues in both countries might serve to clarify the field.

The Issue of Recovery. In recent years, some writers have tended to talk about "recovery" from mental illness (Anthony, 1992) in a way that glosses over the realities of major mental illness. The proponents of this view believe that "much of the chronicity in severe mental illness is due to the way the mental health system and society treat mental illness and not the nature of the illness itself" (Anthony, 1992, p. 1). This point of view has had considerable appeal to many.

The proponents of the use of the word *recovery* are careful to add a disclaimer that they are not claiming that what is after all a biological illness can be cured. Rather, they say that recovery means regaining control over one's life and leading a useful, satisfying life even though symptoms may recur. Such an outlook contains the optimism that is so important in rehabilitation.

However, there is the danger that for many, the word *recovery* does imply cure and that its use may even lead to denial of illness and rejection of needed treatment and rehabilitation. One alternative is to refer instead to *remission*, which can be stable and long lasting. Another alternative is that used by alcoholics who refer to themselves as *recovering* but never as *recovered*, even though it may have been many years since their last drink.

Conclusion

In the past half-century, we have witnessed tremendous progress in the development of the field of psychiatric rehabilitation. We have a well-thought-out philosophy and conceptual underpinnings that enable us to understand what we are doing and why we are doing it. We have models of psychiatric rehabilitation that have been proven effective. We also experience some important and unresolved conceptual and technological differences. But whatever positions are taken on these issues, we do have consensus about what is perhaps the most important issue: that psychiatric rehabilitation is effective and that it should be made available to every person with long-term severe mental illness.

References

Allen, C. I., Gillespie, C. R., and Hall, J. N. "A Comparison of Practices, Attitudes, and Interactions in Two Established Units for People with Psychiatric Disability." *Psychological Medicine*, 1989, *19*, 459–467.

Anderson, C. M., Reiss, D. J., and Hogarty, G. E. *Schizophrenia and the Family*. New York: Guilford Press, 1986.

Anthony, W. A. *The Principles of Psychiatric Rehabilitation*. Baltimore, Md.: University Park Press, 1980.

Anthony, W. A. "Editorial. *Innovations and Research*, 1992, *1*, 1.

Anthony, W. A., Cohen, M. R., and Cohen, B. F. "Psychiatric Rehabilitation." In J. A. Talbott (ed.), *The Chronic Mental Patient: Five Years Later*. Philadelphia: Grune & Stratton, 1984.

Anthony, W. A., and Liberman, R. P. "The Practice of Psychiatric Rehabilitation: Historical, Conceptual, and Research Base." *Schizophrenia Bulletin*, 1986, *12*, 542–559.

Bachrach, L. L. "Psychosocial Rehabilitation and Psychiatry in the Care of Long-Term Patients." *American Journal of Psychiatry*, 1992, *149*, 1455–1463.

Beard, J. H. "Psychiatric Rehabilitation at Fountain House." In J. Meislen (ed.), *Rehabilitation Medicine and Psychiatry*. Springfield, Ill.: Thomas, 1976.

Beard, J. H., Goertzel, V., and Pearce, A. J. "The Effectiveness of Activity Group Therapy with Chronically Regressed Adult Schizophrenics." *International Journal of Group Psychotherapy*, 1958, *8*, 123–136.

Beard, J. H., Propst, R. N., and Malamud, T. J. "The Fountain House Model of Psychiatric Rehabilitation." *Psychosocial Rehabilitation Journal*, 1982, *5*, 47–53.

Beers, C. W. *A Mind That Found Itself*. White Plains, N.Y.: Longman, 1908.

Bellack, A. S., and Mueser, K. T. "Psychosocial Treatment for Schizophrenia." *Schizophrenia Bulletin*, 1993, *19*, 317–336.

Bierer, J. *The Day Hospital: An Experiment in Social Psychiatry and Syntoanalytic Psychotherapy*. London: Lewis, 1951.

Bockoven, J. S. *Moral Treatment in American Psychiatry*. New York: Springer, 1963.

Borus, J. F. "Chronic Mental Patients." In R. Michaels and others (eds.), *Psychiatry*. Philadelphia: Lippincott, 1987.

Braff, D. L., and others. "The Generalized Pattern of Neuropsychological Deficits in Outpatients with Chronic Schizophrenia with Heterogeneous Wisconsin Card Sorting Test Results." *Archives of General Psychiatry*, 1991, *48*, 891–898.

Brown, G. W., Bone, M., Dalison, B., and Wing, J. K. *Schizophrenia and Social Care*. New York: Oxford University Press, 1966.

Cameron, D. E. "The Day Hospital." *Modern Hospital*, 1947, *69*, 60–62.

Carty, R. C., and Breault, G. C. "Geel: A Comprehensive Community Mental Health Program." *Perspectives in Psychiatric Care*, 1967, *5*, 281–285.

Cohen, M. R., Danley, K., and Nemec, P. *Psychiatric Rehabilitation Trainer Packages: Direct Skills Teaching*. Boston: Boston University Center for Psychiatric Rehabilitation, 1986.

Davis, J. M. "Overview: Maintenance Therapy in Psychiatry: I. Schizophrenia." *American Journal of Psychiatry*, 1975, *132*, 1237–1245.

Davis, J. M., and others. "Important Issues in the Drug Treatment of Schizophrenia." *Schizophrenia Bulletin*, 1980, *6*, 70–87.

Deutsch, A. "The History of Mental Hygiene." In J. K. Hall, G. Zilboorg, and H. A. Bunker (eds.), *One Hundred Years of American Psychiatry*. New York: Columbia University Press, 1944.

Dincin, J. "Psychiatric Rehabilitation." *Schizophrenia Bulletin*, 1975, *13*, 131–147.

Dzhagarov, M. A. [Experience in organizing a day hospital for mental patients]. *Nevrophathologia i Psikhiatria*, 1937, *6*, 137–147.

Falloon, I.R.H., and others. "Family Management in the Prevention of Morbidity of Schizophrenia: Clinical Outcome of a Two-Year Longitudinal Study." *Archives of General Psychiatry*, 1985, *42*, 887–896.

Golstein, M. J. (ed.). *New Developments in Interventions with Families of Schizophrenics*. New Directions for Mental Health Services, no. 12. San Francisco: Jossey-Bass, 1981.

Greenblatt, M. Foreword. In B. M. Kramer (ed.), *Day Hospital: A Study of Partial Hospitalization in Psychiatry*. Philadelphia: Grune & Stratton, 1962.

Grob, G. *Mental Institutions in America: Social Policy to 1875*. New York: Free Press, 1973.

Hamilton, S. W. "The History of American Mental Hospitals." In J. K. Hall, G. Zilboorg, and H. A. Bunker (eds.), *One Hundred Years of American Psychiatry*. New York: Columbia University Press, 1944.

Henisz, J. E. *Psychotherapeutic Management in the Day Program*. Springfield, Ill.: Thomas, 1984.

Kane, J. M., and Lieberman, J. A. "Maintenance Pharmacology in Schizophrenia." In H. Y. Meltzer (ed.), *Psychopharmacology: The Third Generation of Progress*. New York: Raven Press, 1987.

Kane, J. M., and Marder, S. R. "Psychopharmacologic Treatment of Schizophrenia." *Schizophrenia Bulletin*, 1993, *19*, 287–302.

Lamb, H. R. "Gearing Day Treatment Centers to Serve Long-Term Patients." In H. R. Lamb and others (eds.), *Community Survival for Long-Term Patients.* San Francisco: Jossey-Bass, 1976.

Lamb, H. R. *Treating the Long-Term Mentally Ill.* San Francisco: Jossey-Bass, 1982.

Lamb, H. R., and Goertzel, V. "Discharged Mental Patients: Are They Really in the Community?" *Archives of General Psychiatry,* 1971, *24,* 29–34.

Lamb, H. R., and Mackota, C. "Vocational Services in a Community Mental Health Program." *Hospital and Community Psychiatry,* 1968, *19,* 315–318.

Lamb, H. R., and others. *Rehabilitation in Community Mental Health.* San Francisco, Jossey-Bass, 1971.

Liberman, R. P. "What Is Schizophrenia?" *Schizophrenia Bulletin,* 1982, *8,* 435–437.

Liberman, R. P. (ed.). *Effective Psychiatric Rehabilitation.* New Directions for Mental Health Services, no. 53. San Francisco: Jossey-Bass, 1992.

Liberman, R. P., DeRisi, W. J., and Mueser, K. T. *Social Skills Training for Psychiatric Patients.* New York: Pergamon Press, 1989.

Liberman, R. P., and Green, M. F. "Whither Cognitive Therapy for Schizophrenia?" *Schizophrenia Bulletin,* 1992, *18,* 27–35.

Liberman, R. P., McCann, M. J., and Wallace, C. J. "Generalization of Behavior Therapy with Psychotics." *British Journal of Psychiatry,* 1976, *129,* 490–496.

Liberman, R. P., and others. *Personal Effectiveness: Guiding People to Assert Feelings and Improve Their Social Skills.* Champaign, Ill.: Research Press, 1975.

Mora, G., and Brand, J. (eds.). *Psychiatry and Its History.* Springfield, Ill.: Thomas, 1970.

Munich, R. L., and Lang, E. "The Boundaries of Psychiatric Rehabilitation." *Hospital and Community Psychiatry,* 1993, *44,* 661–665.

Neuchterlein, K. H., and Dawson, M. E. "A Heuristic Vulnerability/Stress Model of Schizophrenic Episodes." *Schizophrenia Bulletin,* 1984a, *10,* 300–312.

Neuchterlein, K. H., and Dawson, M. E. "Information Processing and Attentional Functioning in the Developmental Course of Schizophrenic Disorders." *Schizophrenia Bulletin,* 1984b, *10,* 160–203.

Olshansky, S. "Some Assumptions Challenged." *Community Mental Health Journal,* 1968, *4,* 153–156.

Paul, G. L., and Lentz, R. J. *Psychosocial Treatment of Chronic Mental Patients: Milieu Versus Social Learning Programs.* Cambridge, Mass.: Harvard University Press, 1977.

Pollock, H. M. *Family Care of Mental Patients.* Utica, N.Y.: State Hospitals Press, 1936.

Rothman, D. *The Discovery of the Asylum: Social Order and Disorder in the New Republic.* New York: Little, Brown, 1971.

Shepherd, G. "Work and Rehabilitation." *Current Opinion in Psychiatry,* 1988, *1,* 217–221.

Shepherd, G. "Psychiatric Rehabilitation in the 1990s." In F. N. Watts and D. H. Bennett (eds.), *Theory and Practice of Psychiatric Rehabilitation.* New York: Wiley, 1991.

Simon, W. B. "On Reluctance to Leave the Public Mental Hospital." *Psychiatry,* 1965, *28,* 145–156.

Wing, J. K. "The Management of Schizophrenia in the Community." Paper presented at the annual meeting of the American College of Psychiatrists, Atlanta, Feb. 1977.

Wing, J. K., and Morris, B. (eds.). *Handbook of Psychiatric Rehabilitation Practice.* New York: Oxford University Press, 1981.

H. Richard Lamb is professor of psychiatry and the behavioral sciences at Keck School of Medicine, University of Southern California, in Los Angeles.

INDEX

Back Issue/Subscription Order Form

Copy or detach and send to:
Jossey-Bass, 350 Sansome Street, San Francisco CA 94104-1342

Call or fax toll free!
Phone 888-378-2537 6AM-5PM PST; Fax 800-605-2665

Back issues: Please send me the following issues at $28 each.
(Important: please include series initials and issue number, such as MHS90.)

1. MHS _____

_____

$ _____ Total for single issues

$ _____ Shipping charges (for single issues *only;* subscriptions are exempt
from shipping charges): Up to $30, add $5^{50} • $30^{01}–$50, add $6^{50}
$50^{01}–$75, add $8 • $75^{01}–$100, add $10 • $100^{01}–$150, add $12
Over $150, call for shipping charge

Subscriptions   Please ❑ start   ❑ renew my subscription to *New Directions for
Mental Health Services* for the year ___ at the following rate:

U.S.:	❑ Individual $66	❑ Institutional $121
Canada:	❑ Individual $66	❑ Institutional $161
All others:	❑ Individual $90	❑ Institutional $195

$ _____ Total single issues and subscriptions (Add appropriate sales tax for
your state for single issue orders. No sales tax for U.S. subscriptions.
Canadian residents, add GST for subscriptions.)

❑ Payment enclosed (U.S. check or money order only)

❑ VISA, MC, AmEx, Discover Card #_____ Exp. date_____

Signature _____ Day phone _____

❑ Bill me (U.S. institutional orders only. Purchase order required.)

Purchase order #_____

Federal Tax ID 135593032   GST 89102-8052

Name _____

Address _____

_____

Phone_____ E-mail _____

For more information about Jossey-Bass, visit our Web site at:
www.josseybass.com   **PRIORITY CODE = ND1**